The Bi...

	SECOND STAGE:	**THIRD STAGE:**
Transition	*PUSHING & BIRTH*	*PLACENTA*

10cm

9cm

8cm

Pant Blow →

Sustained Pushing
or Gentle Pushing →

The Birth Book

by Heather Moll

Illustrations by Heidi Schultz

Publisher's Cataloging-in-Publication data

Names: Moll, Heather, author | Schultz, Heidi, illustrator.
Title: The Birth book / by Heather Moll ; illustrations by Heidi Schultz.
Description: McMinnville, Oregon: Kendall Dean Publishing, 2015.
Identifiers: ISBN: 978-0-9969923-0-5 | LCCN: 2015918797
Subjects: LCSH: Pregnancy | Childbirth. | BISAC: HEALTH & FITNESS / Pregnancy & Childbirth.
Classification: LCC: RG525 .M545 2015 | DDC: 618.2--dc23.

ISBN 978-0-9969923-0-5

The information in this book should not be treated as a substitute for professional medical advice; always consult a medical practitioner. This book is in no way intended to replace, supercede or conflict with the advice given by your own doctor. The ultimate decision concerning care should be made between you and your care provider. We strongly recommend you follow his or her advice. The information in this book is general and is offered with no guarantees on the part of the author or publisher. Neither the author nor the publisher can be held responsible for any loss, claim or damage arising out of the use (or misuse) of the information in this book or the failure to take medical advice. Always consult your medical professional.

Editing, Book Design and Project Management by Jeremy Moll

First Edition

Printed and bound by Friesens in Canada.
First printed in December 2015.

Published by Kendall Dean Publishing LLC

www.TheBirthBook.com

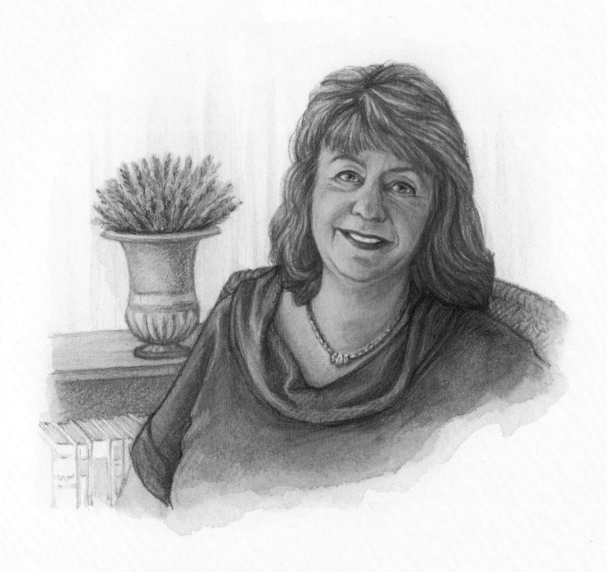

Contained in this book is the wisdom and experience acquired during a 30-year career delivering 950 babies and teaching childbirth classes to over 18,000 expectant parents.

When I tell women I am a midwife, many begin to share the story of the birth of their children. Some stories are positive and some are negative, but all are remembered in vivid detail.

When you tell your birth story, I want it to be a good one.

That is my wish for you. Learn this data. Study it well.

Love,

Heather Moll

Heather Moll, author

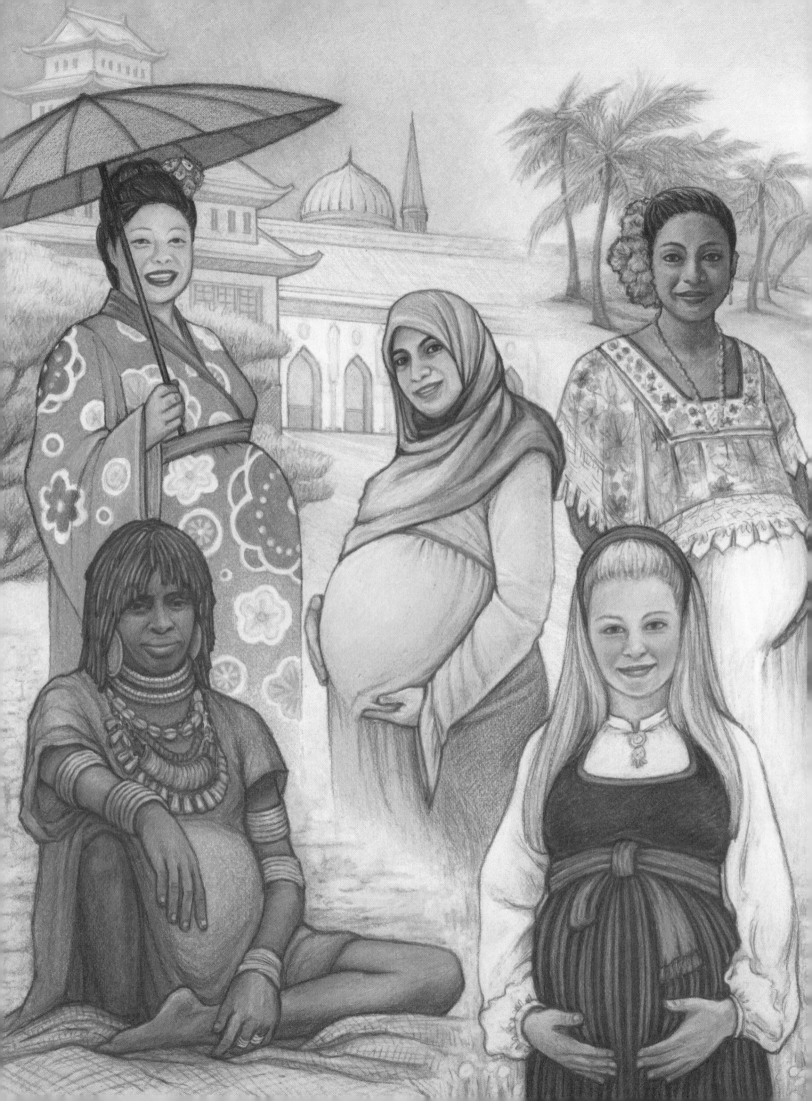

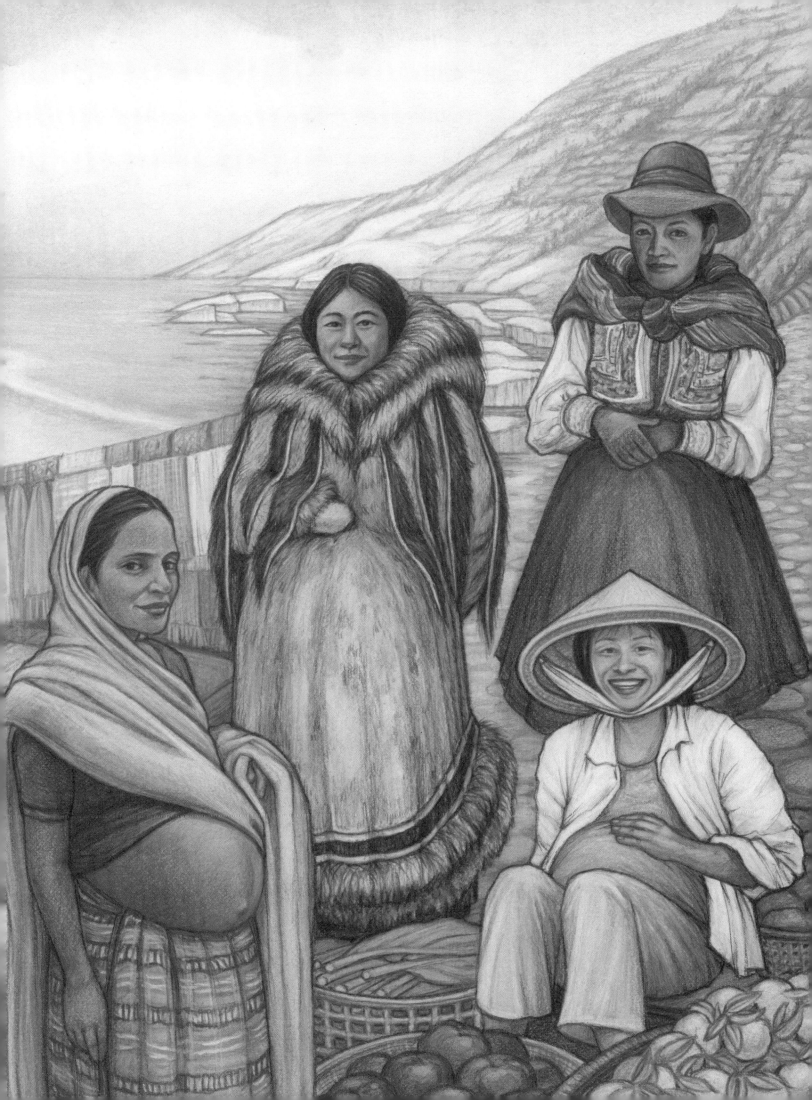

TABLE OF CONTENTS

CHILDBIRTH EXPLAINED 1

What Is Childbirth? 3

The Pregnant Body 4

Contractions: The Activity of Labor 7

Before Labor Begins 9

Labor Begins 13

The Stages of Labor 14

   First Stage of Labor: Dilation 16

      Early Labor 19

      Active Labor 21

      Transition 23

      Note: Effacement 27

   Second Stage of Labor: Pushing and Birth 28

      Pushing 33

         The Baby's Journey Through the Pelvis 34

         Note: Head Station 36

         Crowning 41

      Birth 42

   Third Stage of Labor: Placenta 63

      Immediate Recovery 68

BASIC LABOR SKILLS 73

Keeping a Labor Log 74

How to Measure Contractions 76

When to Go to the Birth Setting 78

Traveling to the Birth Setting 81

Creating Your Birth Setting 83

The Basic Labor Strategy 84

Labor Techniques 87

   Breathing Techniques 89

   Labor Positions 90

      The Importance of Walking 97

Comfort Techniques 98

Managing Pain in Labor 105
How to Move a Woman in Labor 106
Labor Fatigue 109

HOW TO GET THROUGH LABOR 111

Early Labor 112
Active Labor 116
Transition 120
   The Premature Urge to Push 124
Pushing 126
Birth 130
   The Newborn Arrives 134
Delivery of Placenta 136

PREPARING FOR LABOR 139

Designing Your Birth Experience 140
   The Birth Environment 142
   Labor Support Team 145
     The Labor Coach 147
   Being Prepared 149
Creating Your Birth Plan 151

THE BIRTH EXPERIENCE 153

CLOSING COMMENTS 187

ADDITIONAL RESOURCES 195

Medical Intervention
Summary of Breathing Techniques
Summary of Labor Positions

CHILDBIRTH EXPLAINED

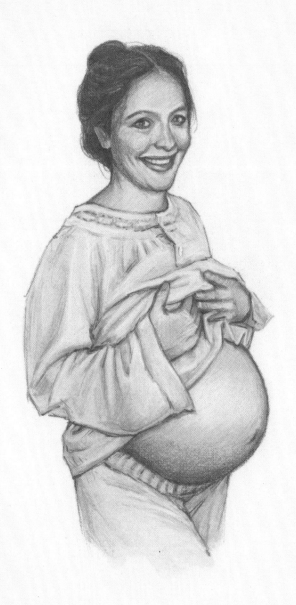

WHAT IS CHILDBIRTH?

Childbirth is the process by which a woman's body moves her baby from her womb into the world.

This process is simple. It is a natural sequence of events created by the body outside of the mother's control.

Every birth is different, but each one follows the same basic principles which can be understood and managed.

THE PREGNANT BODY

Uterus

The uterus is an organ made of very strong muscles. Its purpose is to provide the environment for the developing baby during pregnancy and to move the baby out of the body during birth.

Cervix

The cervix is the opening of the uterus. During pregnancy, it is closed and holds the baby inside. During labor, the uterus pulls the cervix open so that the baby can pass through.

Mucus Plug

During pregnancy, the cervix is sealed with a plug of mucus. This plug will come out early in the labor process.

Placenta

The placenta is a temporary organ which connects the growing baby to its mother. The placenta's role is to provide oxygen and nutrients to the developing baby. It is attached to the wall of the uterus. After the baby is born, the placenta detaches and is pushed out of the mother's body.

Umbilical Cord

The umbilical cord connects the developing baby to the placenta.

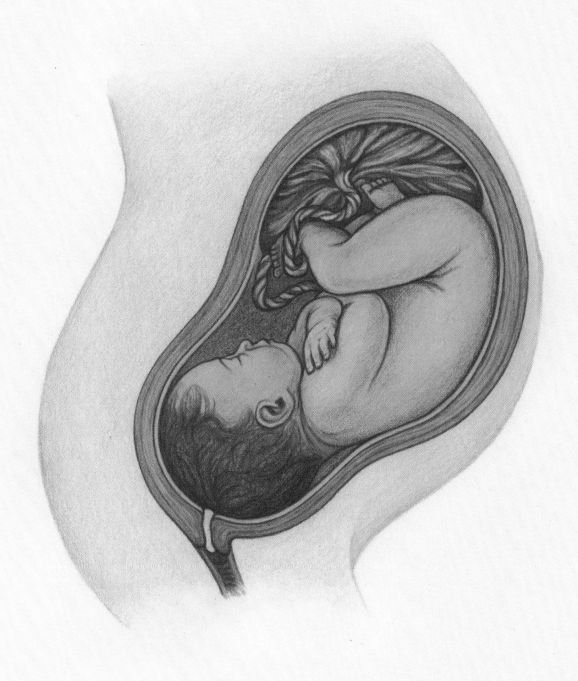

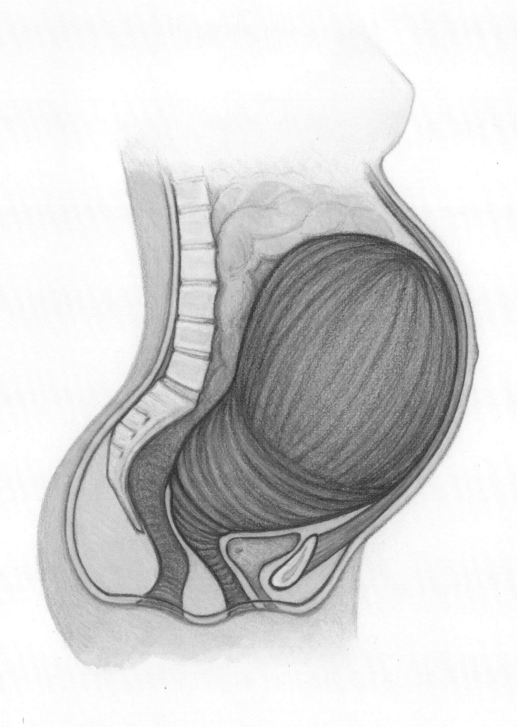

CONTRACTIONS
The Activity of Labor

The role of the uterus during labor is to pull itself open and to push the baby out of the mother's body. It does this by pulling its muscles tight for a minute or so at a time and then by pausing to take a rest.

A single instance of the uterus pulling with its muscles is called a "contraction".

The labor process is a long series of repeating contractions which results in the birth of the baby.

As labor progresses, the contractions get stronger, longer and more frequent.

Contractions happen independently from the mother's control. Mother Nature designed it so that they occur no matter how she feels about it.

In other words, the laboring mother does not "think up her contractions."

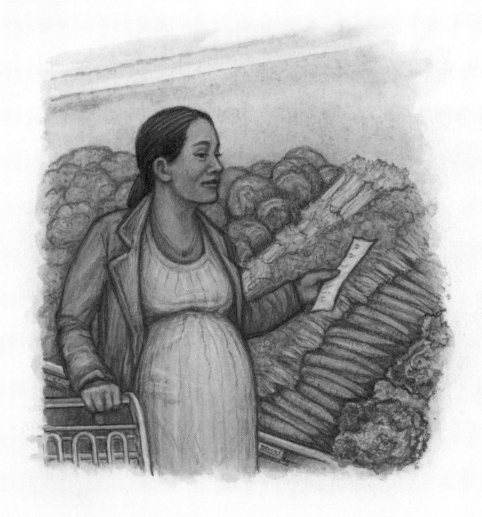

BEFORE LABOR BEGINS

In the weeks leading up to the labor, the mother's body is undergoing its final preparations for the birth of the baby.

Despite the discomforts of late pregnancy, this preparation stage is important as two vital things are happening.

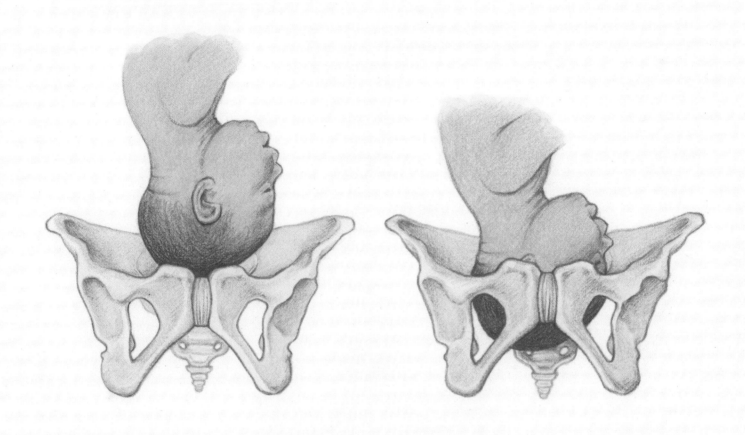

The baby is moving deeper into the pelvis.

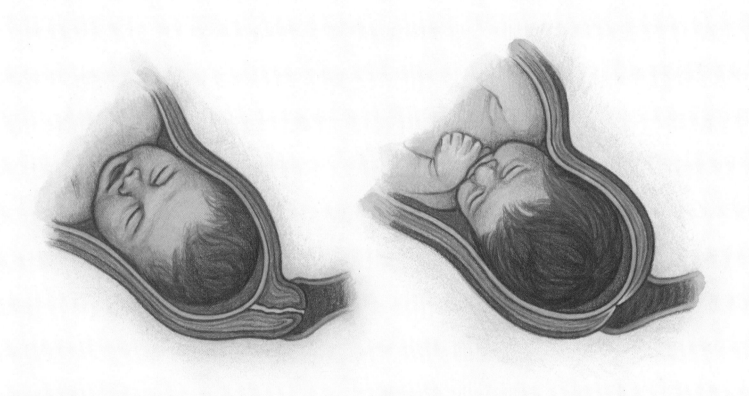

The cervix is beginning to thin and soften.

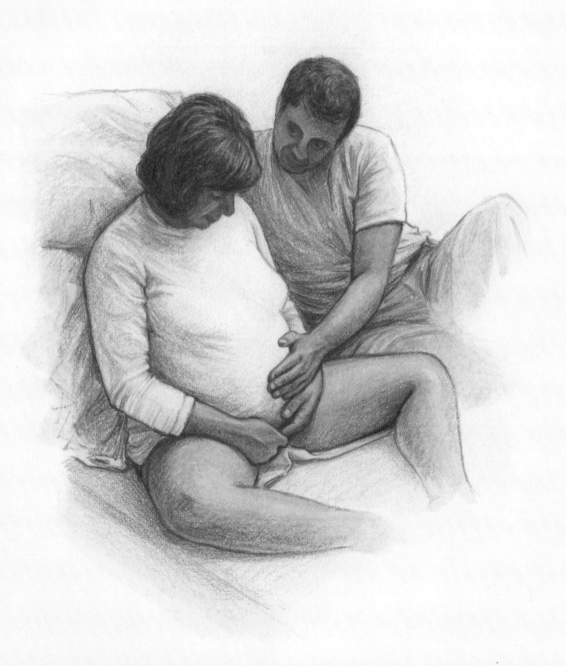

LABOR BEGINS

The labor process is a long sequence of contractions which results in the birth of the baby.

This process usually does not begin suddenly; it begins gradually.

Labor has begun when contractions have settled into a repeating pattern and are not stopping.

THE STAGES OF LABOR

The entire birth process happens in three stages.

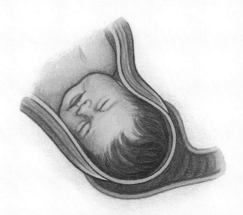

First Stage of Labor:
Dilation

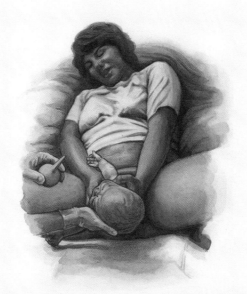

Second Stage of Labor:
Pushing and Birth

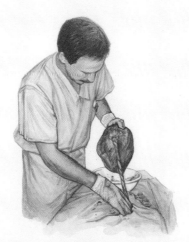

Third Stage of Labor:
Delivery of the Placenta

FIRST STAGE OF LABOR

Dilation

The word "dilate" means "to open or widen".

During the First Stage of Labor, the uterus dilates the cervix fully open to 10 centimeters.

This stage of labor has three parts.

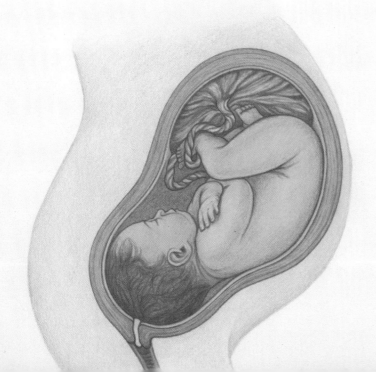

First Stage   Second Stage   Third Stage

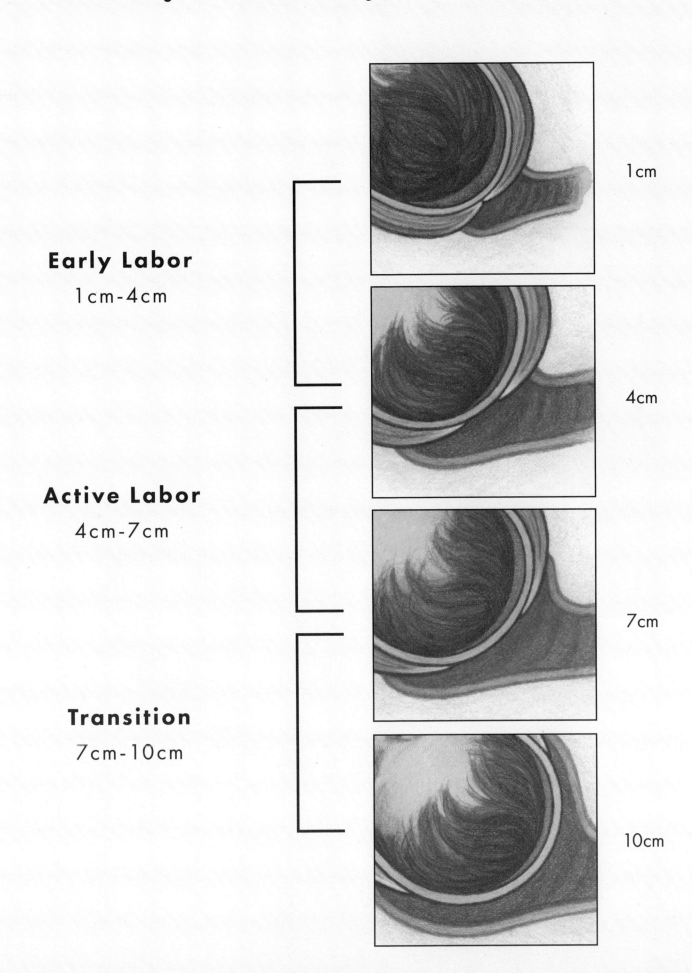

Early Labor
1cm-4cm

Active Labor
4cm-7cm

Transition
7cm-10cm

1cm

4cm

7cm

10cm

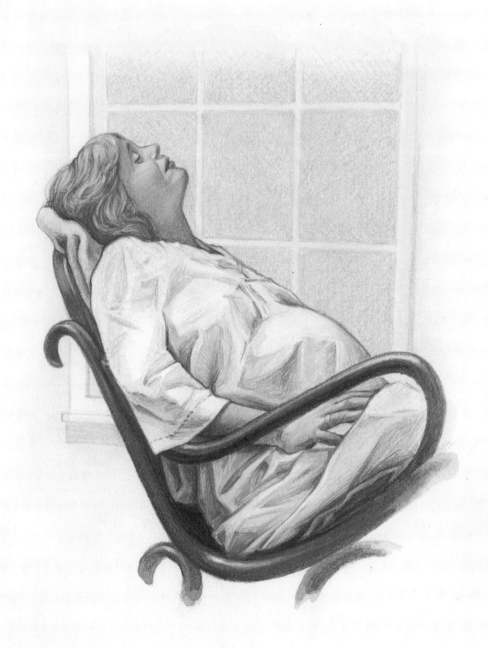

Early Labor

During Early Labor, the uterus dilates the cervix to 4cm.

Usually the mother settles into the process at home until it is time to go to the birth setting for the rest of labor.

1cm

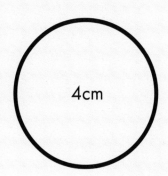

4cm

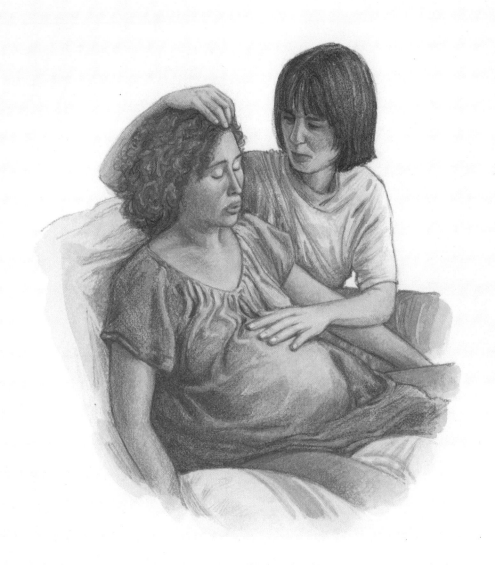

Active Labor

During Active Labor, the uterus dilates the cervix to 7 cm.

The contractions are now more powerful and more frequent.

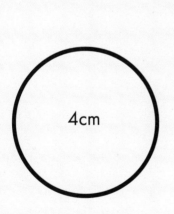

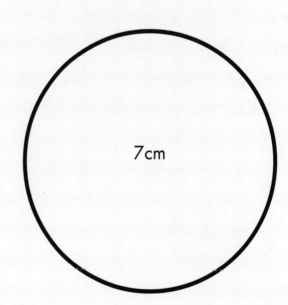

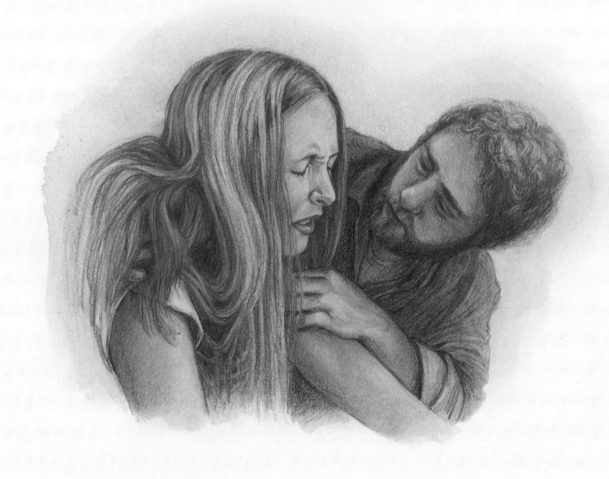

Transition

During Transition, the uterus completes the dilation of the cervix by opening it to 10 centimeters.

The Transition phase is famous for its strength and intensity.

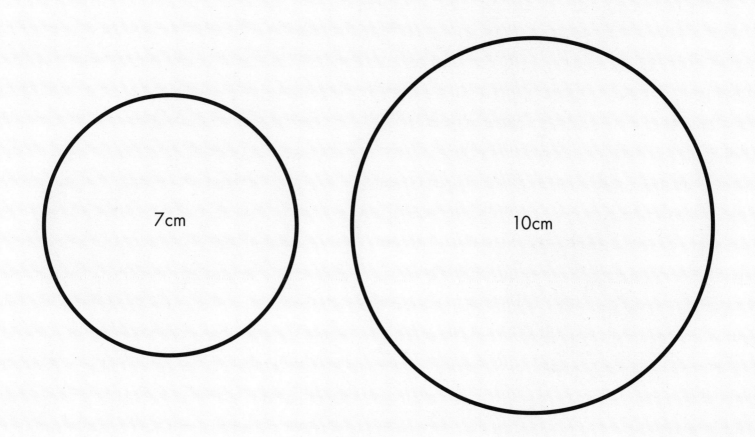

The First Stage of Labor is complete when the cervix is fully dilated to 10 centimeters.

"It's like going from the cheerio to the bagel."

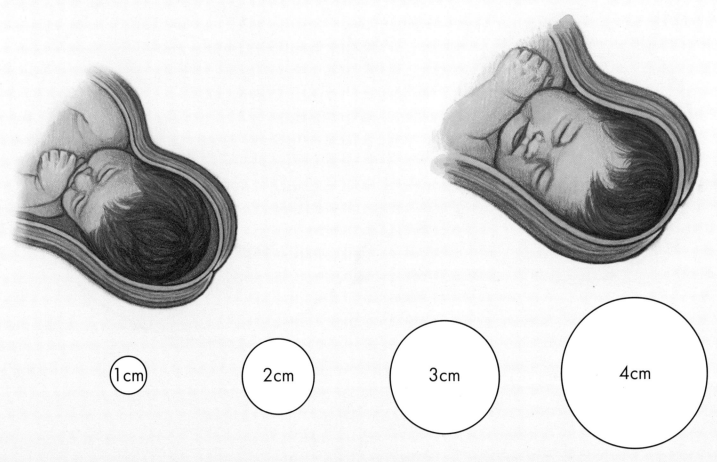

1cm   2cm   3cm   4cm

First Stage   Second Stage   Third Stage

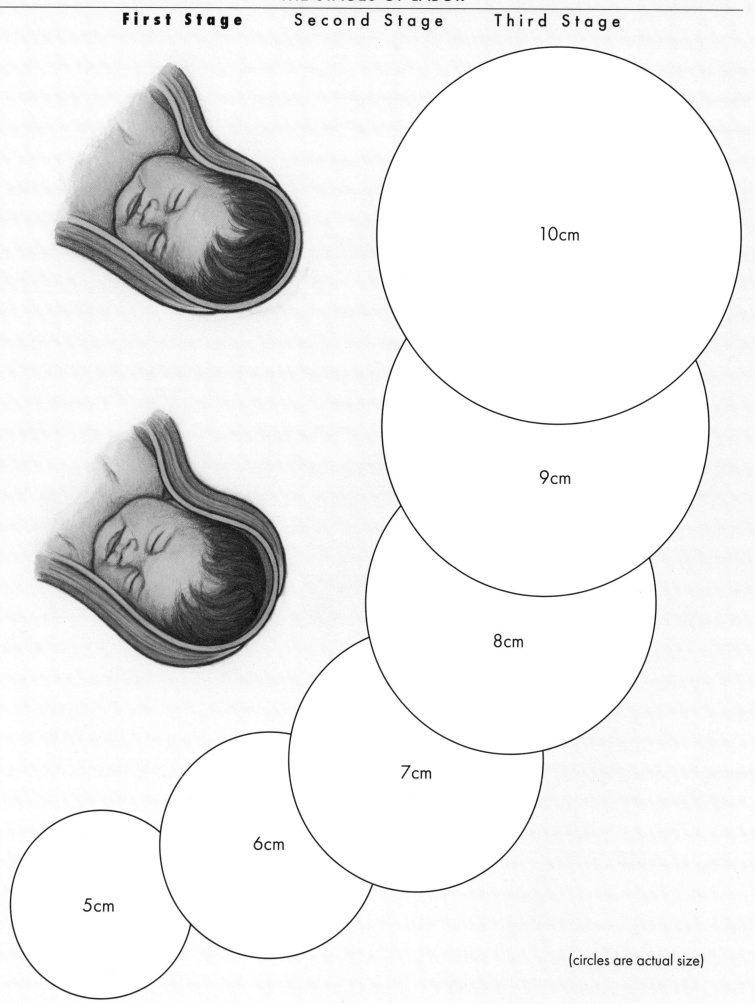

10cm

9cm

8cm

7cm

6cm

5cm

(circles are actual size)

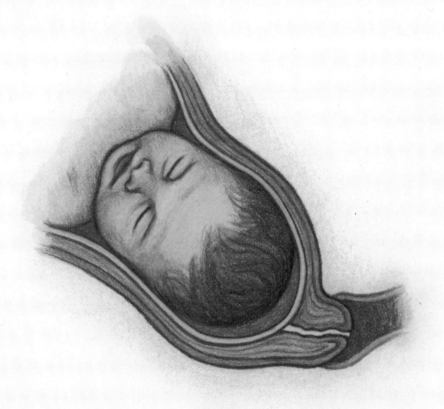

a thick and closed cervix

NOTE: In order for the cervix to fully dilate, it must first thin and soften.

This thinning and softening of the cervix is called "effacement".

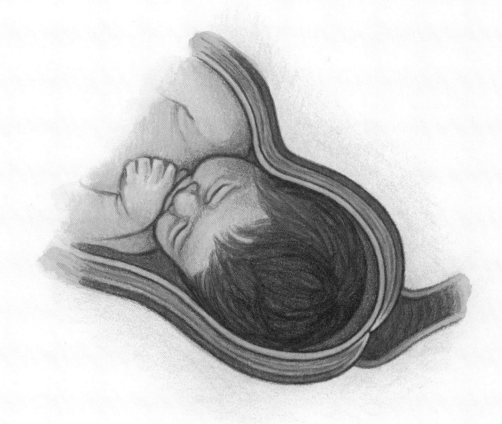

a fully effaced cervix

SECOND STAGE OF LABOR

Pushing and Birth

In the Second Stage of Labor, the mother pushes along with the contractions of the uterus to move the baby down through the birth canal and out of her body.

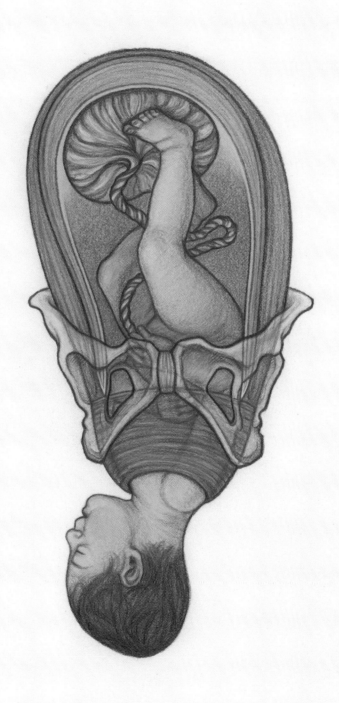

The Second Stage of Labor has two phases.

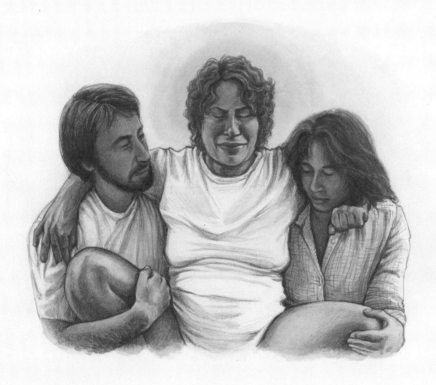

Pushing

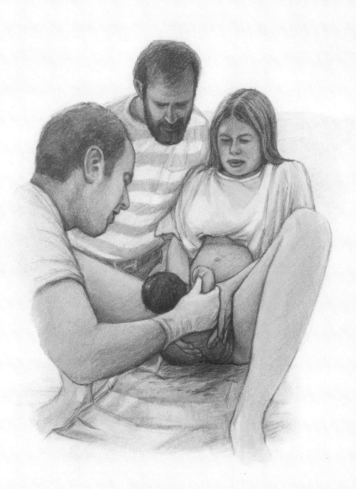

Birth

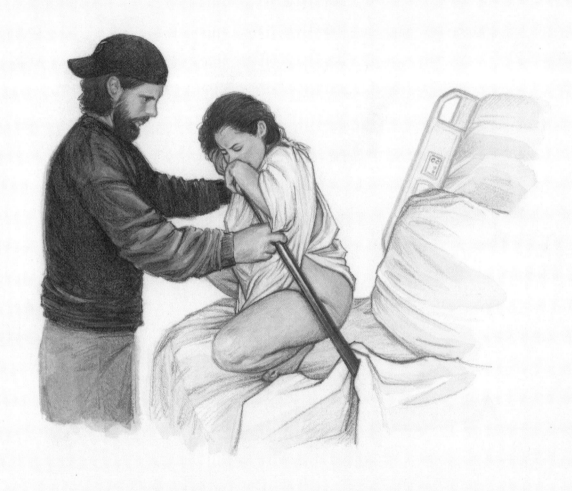

Pushing

Once the cervix is fully dilated, the mother begins to push along with the contractions of the uterus to move the baby down the birth canal until the baby's head is visible from the outside.

The Baby's Journey Through the Pelvis

In order for the baby to fit through the pelvis on its way down the birth canal, its head must go through a series of rotations.

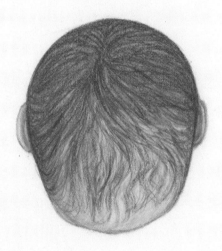

The baby's head is widest from front to back.

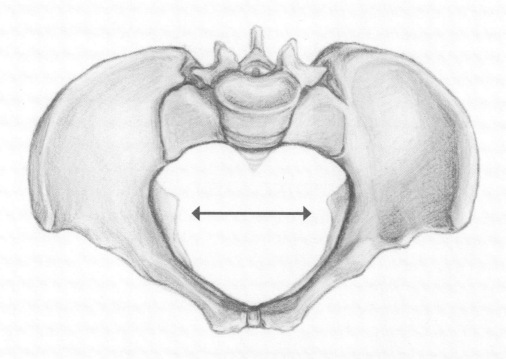

The top opening of the pelvis is widest from side to side.

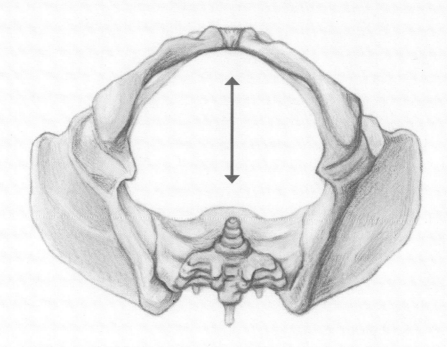

The bottom opening of the pelvis, however, is widest from top to bottom.

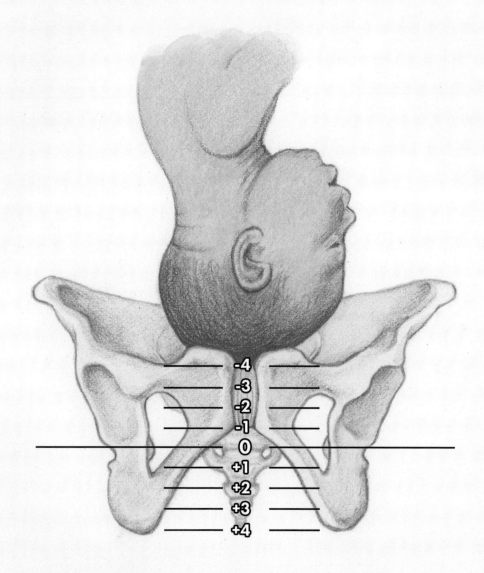

NOTE: The baby's downward progress through the pelvis is measured in "head station".

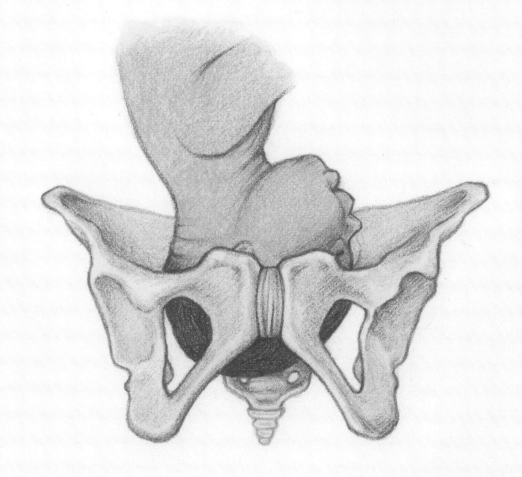

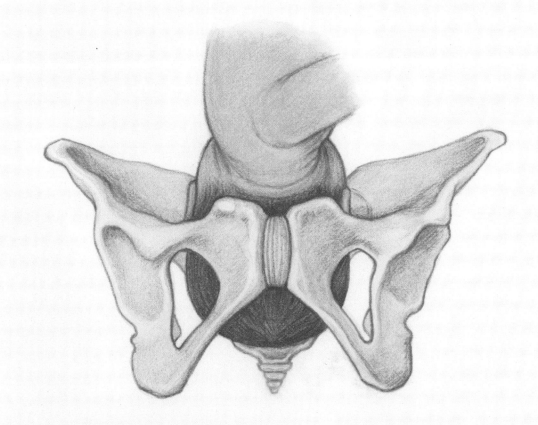

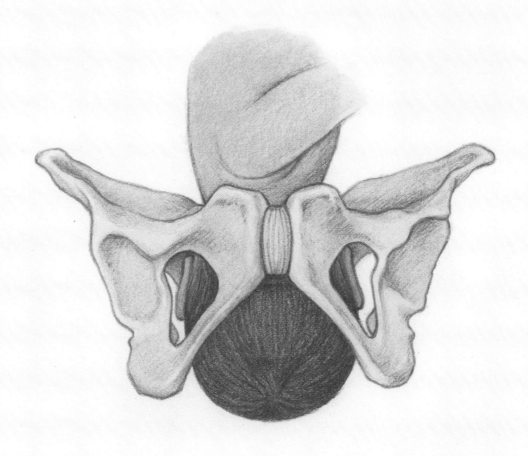

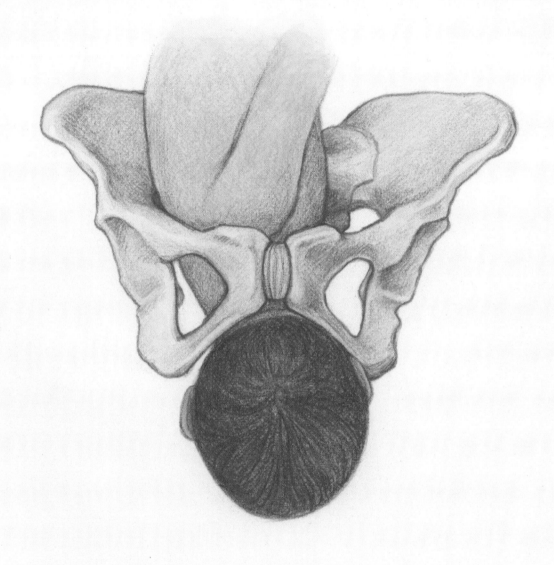

Crowning

Eventually the head will reach the "crowning position". This means that the head is now visible from the outside.

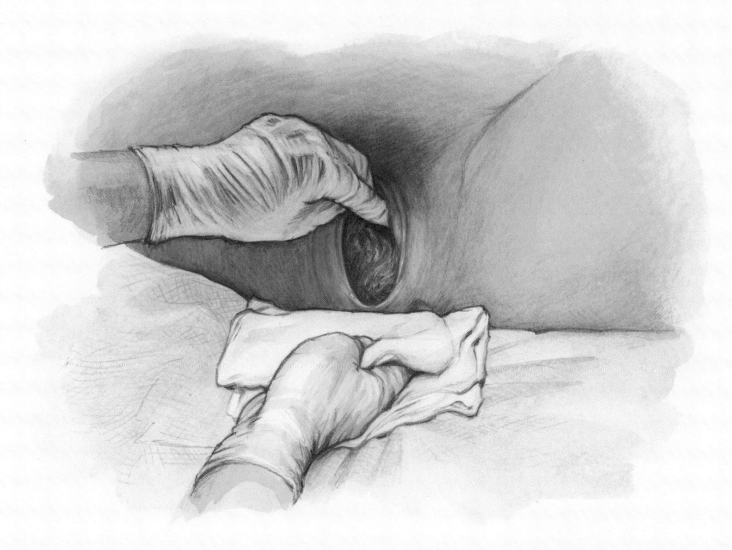

Birth

Once the crowning position is reached, the mother is guided by her care provider to push gently to allow the tissues of the vagina to expand. Birth of the baby occurs within just a few contractions.

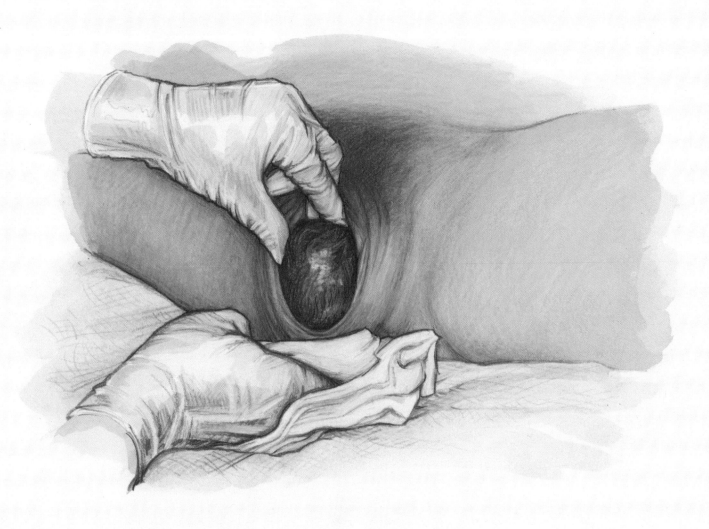

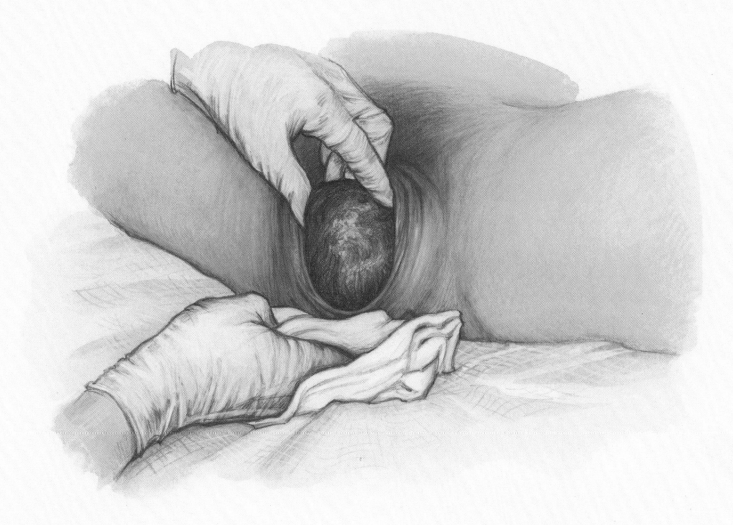

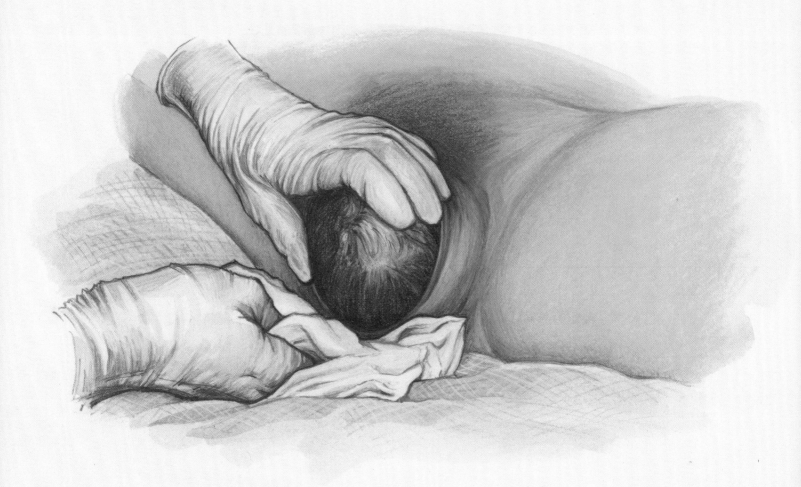

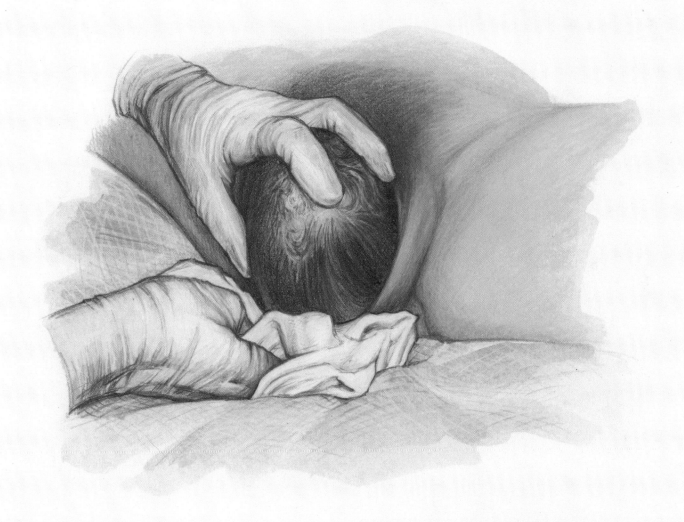

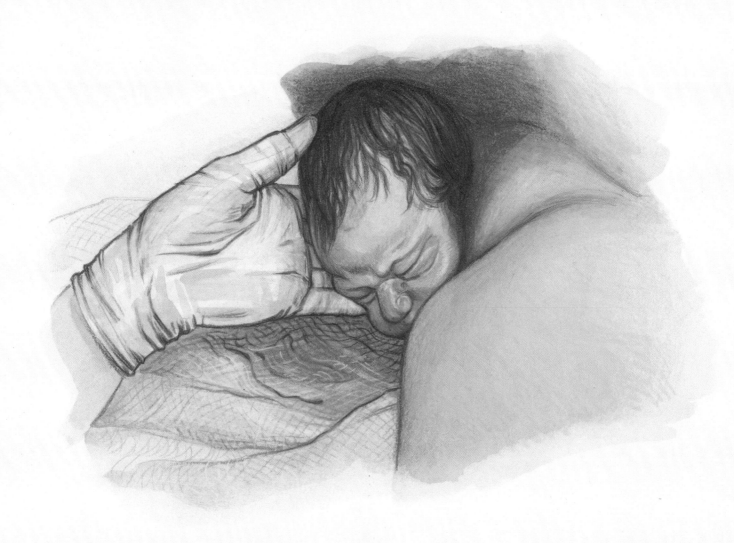

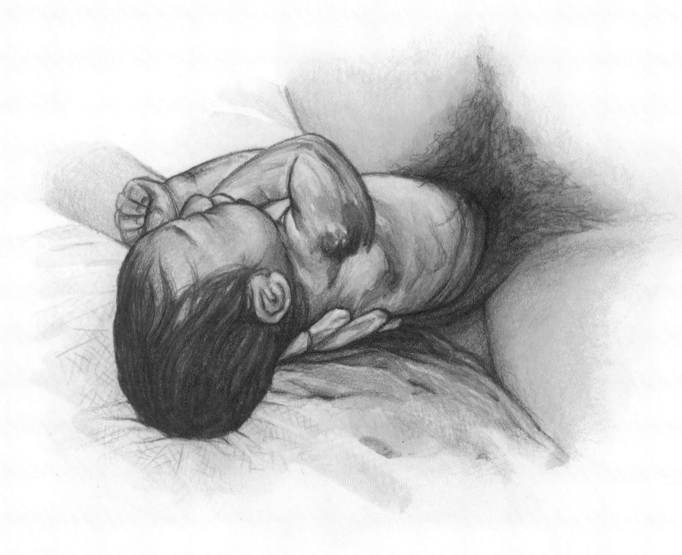

Once the baby's head is delivered, the rest of the body comes out easily.

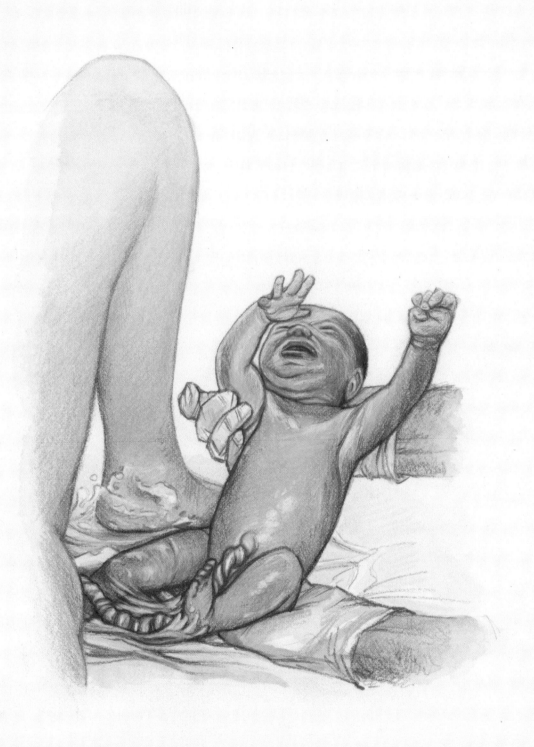

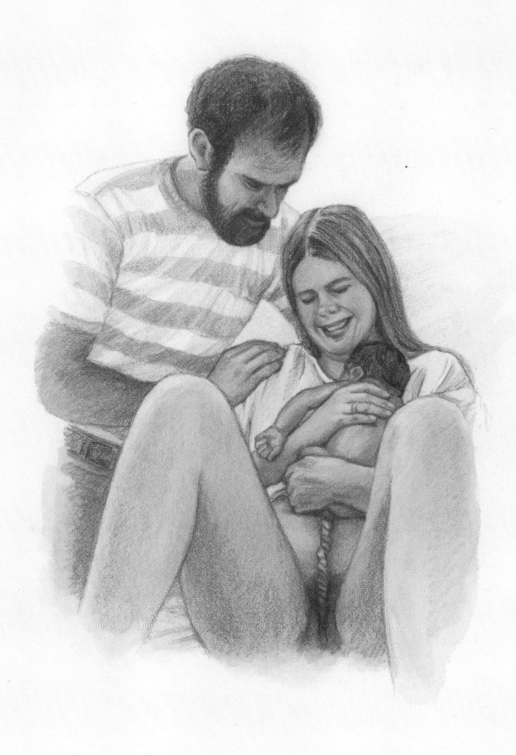

The baby will fill its lungs with air for the first time.

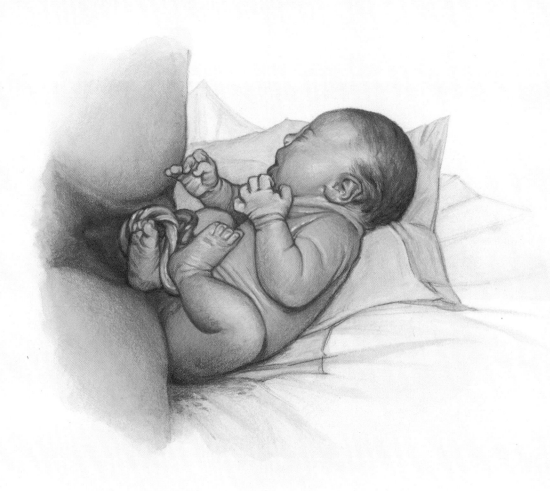

First Stage　　**Second Stage**　　Third Stage

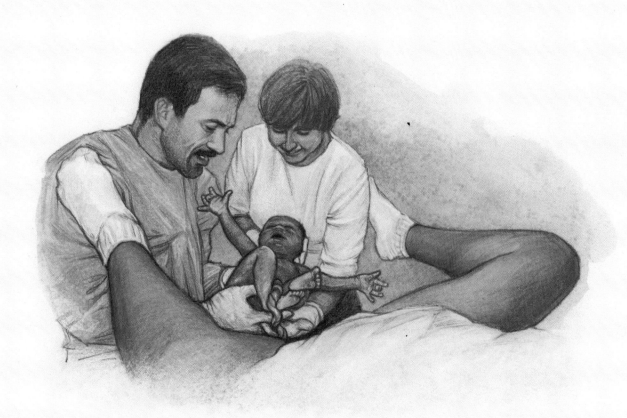

Within minutes, the baby will transition to its own life support system, one of nature's most complex and miraculous feats. The baby no longer needs the umbilical cord connection. The pulsating cord begins to constrict and turn white as the flow of blood from the placenta through the cord reduces.

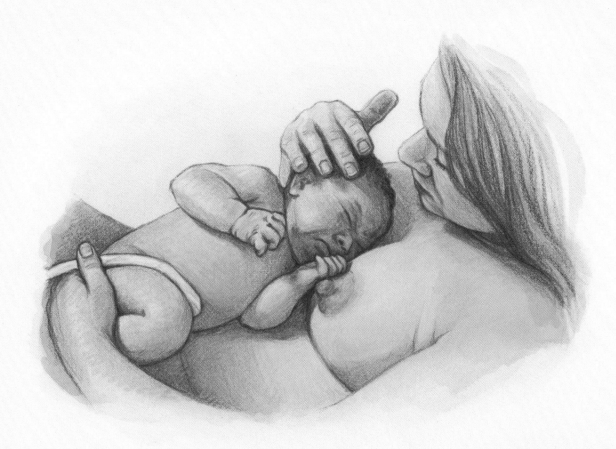

After the cord stops pulsating, the care provider will clamp it. The labor partner is often given the opportunity to cut the cord.

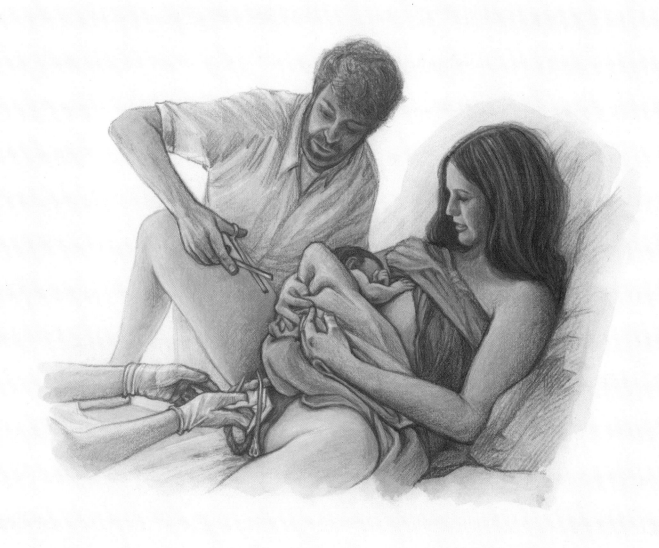

The baby will be covered with a warm blanket while recovering from the immediate moment of birth. Its color may look a bit bluish, but this will turn more pink within a few minutes.

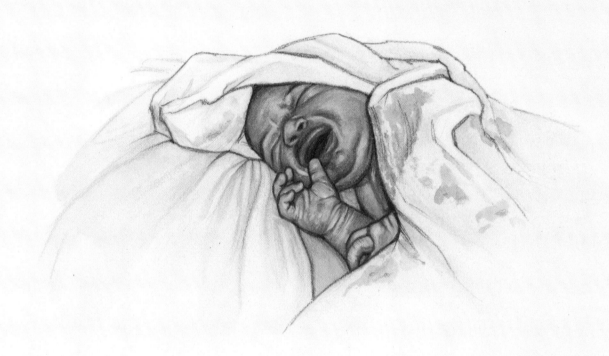

Often a newborn's head may look elongated. A baby's head molds to accommodate the pressure of the birth canal. The head will regain its normal shape within a couple of hours.

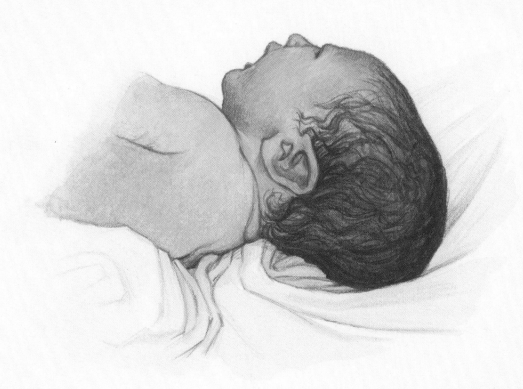

First Stage   **Second Stage**   Third Stage

The new baby may also look sort of "mushed" with a smashed nose, folded ears and puffy eyes. This is normal and is caused by the tremendous amount of pressure exerted on the baby during labor. The baby's appearance will improve soon after its birth.

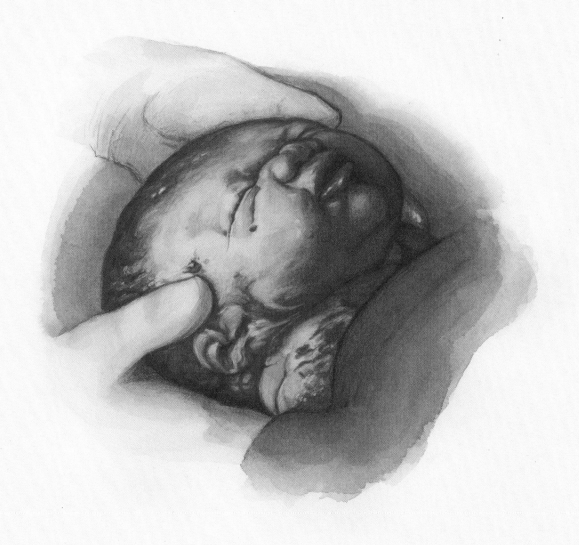

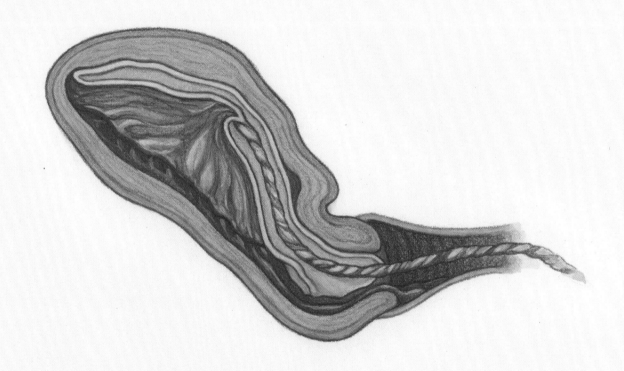

THIRD STAGE OF LABOR

Placenta

Within a few minutes after the birth of the baby, the uterus will begin to contract again to separate the placenta from the wall of the uterus and to push it out of the body.

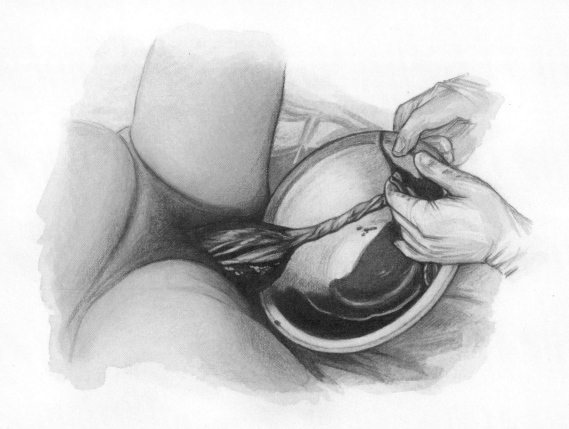

The care provider will pull gently on the cord to guide the placenta out of the mother's body.

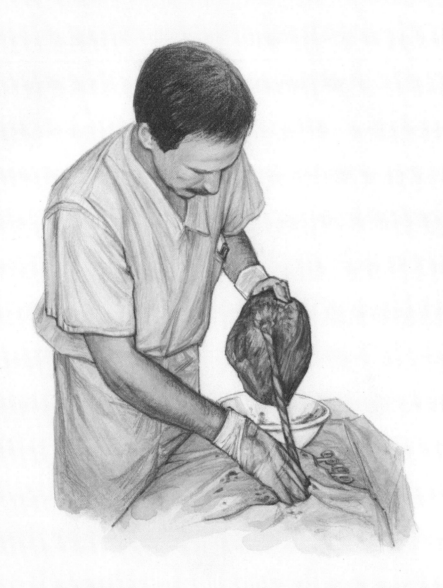

The doctor will examine the placenta after the birth to ensure the detachment from the uterus was complete. He will also check to see that the formation of the placenta is normal.

Immediate Recovery

The detachment of the placenta exposes blood vessels in the wall of the uterus which were used for the baby's support during pregnancy.

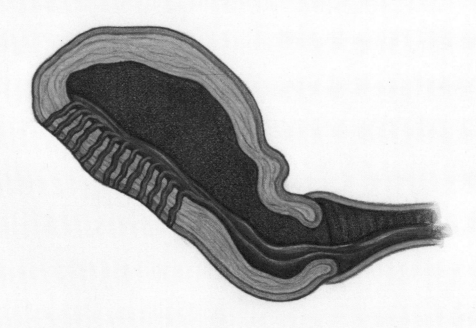

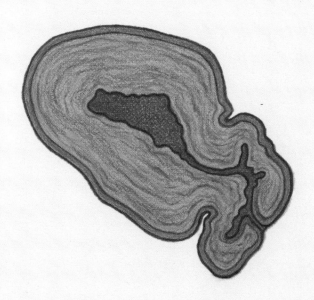

The uterus will contract and squeeze itself closed
to control the bleeding. It will continue to do this
for several weeks while the uterus heals.

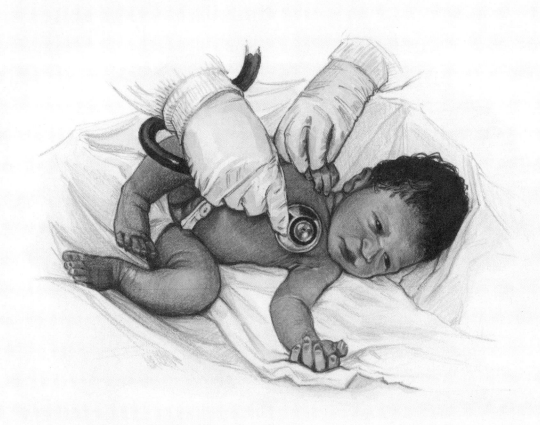

After the placenta is delivered, the care provider will examine the newborn to ensure the baby is healthy and recovering well from the birth process.

BASIC LABOR SKILLS

Keeping a Labor Log

When signs of labor begin, it is a good idea to have your labor coach keep a labor log for the remainder of the birth. It will help you answer important questions asked by your care provider during labor. It also provides a journal on the history of your labor for you to look back on later.

Significant events should be recorded along with the time they occurred.

Labor Log entries can include:

- measurement of contractions
- dilation progress
- bloody discharge
- leaking fluid
- medical procedures done
- newborn's birth time and vital statistics upon its birth

The labor log should be simple and should not become a distraction. You will likely find this tool very useful.

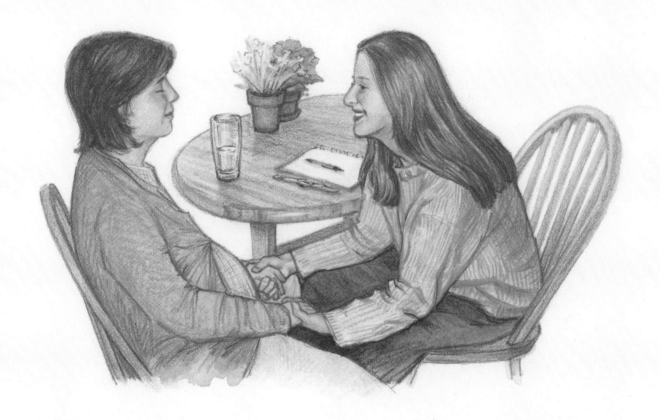

Keeping a Labor Log

How to Measure Contractions

Remember that the labor process is a long series of repeating contractions which results in the birth of the baby. Measuring the frequency, length and strength of them is very useful in determining the overall progress of the labor.

Take the following measurements for 20 or 30 minutes every few hours, and record them in your labor log.

Frequency: The amount of time between the beginning of a contraction and the beginning of the next.

Length: The amount of time the uterus stays tightened up during a contraction.

Strength: How strongly the muscles are contracting. You can come up with your own measurement system, such as a scale of 1-10.

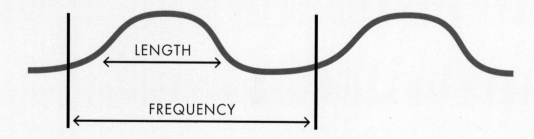

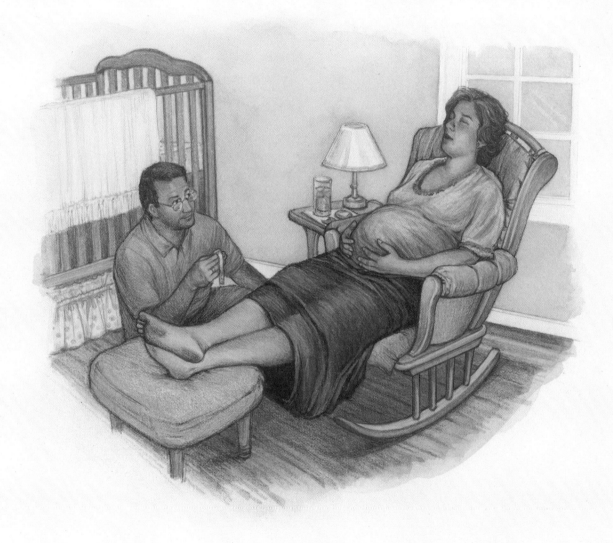

When to Go to the Birth Setting

The time to go to the birth setting is when labor (and not false labor) has begun. Therefore, it's important to know the difference between false labor and labor.

NOTE: Final confirmation that it's time to go to the birth setting comes from a conversation with your care provider.

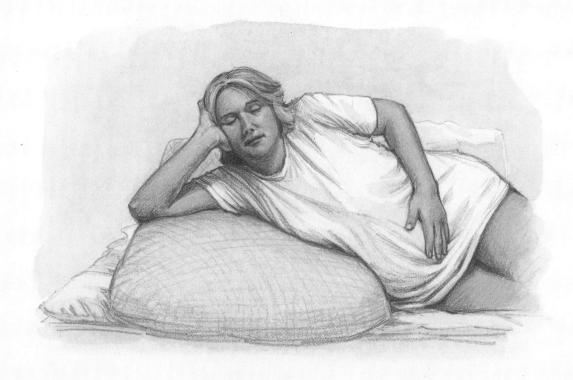

SIGNS OF FALSE LABOR

- Contractions are not settling into a pattern

- Contractions do not seem to be getting stronger

- Moving around or changing positions seems to make contractions lessen in strength

- The tightening of the uterus does not seem to have a definite beginning or ending point

SIGNS OF LABOR

- Contractions are beginning to occur in a regular pattern

- Contractions have a definite beginning and end

- Contractions are beginning every five minutes or less

- Contractions are lasting 60 seconds or longer

- The mother is having a difficult time talking or walking during a contraction

- Contractions are not stopping even though the mother is moving or changing positions

- This has been happening for more than an hour

NOTE: Always inform your care provider if you experience any leaking fluid.

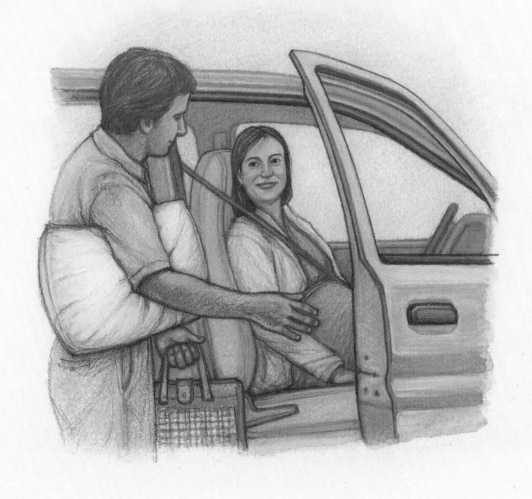

Traveling to the Birth Setting

In most cases, labor begins gradually. There is no need to rush or panic. It may take several hours of contractions and a conversation with your care provider to finally decide to depart for your birth setting.

While traveling to the birth setting be safe, take your time and take steps to ensure her comfort.

You can use extra bed pillows to make her car ride more comfortable, as she will be having contractions on the way.

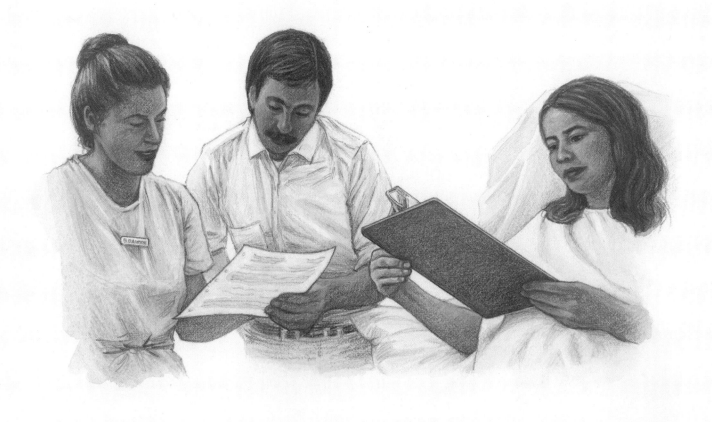

Creating Your Birth Setting

When you arrive at the birth setting, the first thing to do is to get settled and to make the environment comfortable and distraction-free. You will be here for the rest of the birth.

Here are some tips for creating a comfortable birth environment:

- adjust lighting so it is soft and dim

- ensure those present are using quiet voices

- arrange labor supplies nearby

- put on soft music or nature sounds

- collect 4-6 extra pillows for labor positions

- have the mother put on comfortable clothing for labor

- meet the medical staff and share your birth plan with them

The Basic Labor Strategy

All throughout the birth process, the basic strategy remains the same:

> **Get through each contraction and use the rest period to relax and prepare for the next one.**

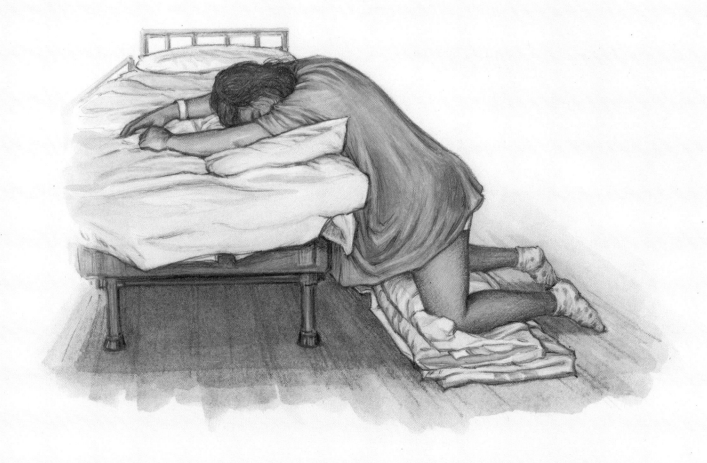

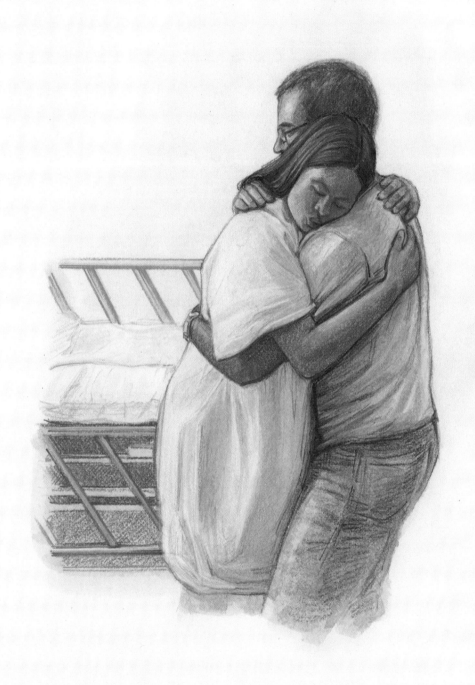

LABOR TECHNIQUES

There are three basic categories of techniques that you will use to get through the contractions of the labor process.

- **Breathing Techniques**
- **Labor Positions**
- **Comfort Techniques**

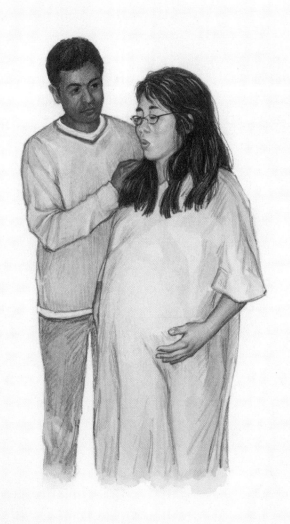

Breathing Techniques

When contractions get painful, the natural response is to tighten up and hold your breath. It is important that you don't do this, however, as it works against what the body is trying to do to deliver the baby.

Each stage of labor has its own suggested breathing techniques to help you work with the contraction rather than against it.

This will ensure the baby continues to receive plenty of oxygen during the compression of the contraction.

Proper breathing also gives you something to focus on <u>doing</u> during the intense and overwhelming sensations of these contractions.

It is important to practice these breathing techniques before labor so that you are familiar with them.

Labor Positions

There are a variety of labor positions for you to choose from to assist in relaxation and comfort and to encourage the descent and rotation of the baby through the pelvis. While a woman may stay in a preferred labor position for several hours, it is still beneficial to change positions often.

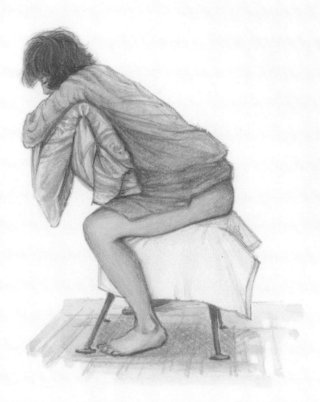

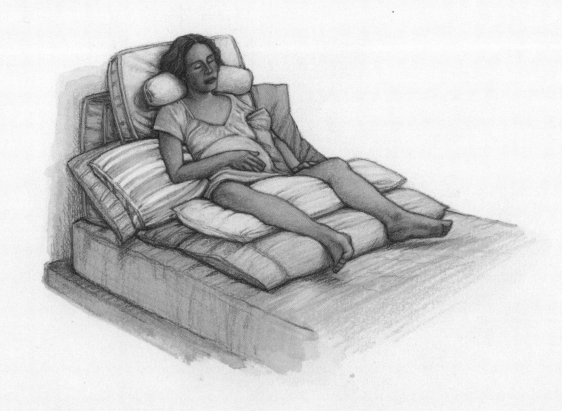

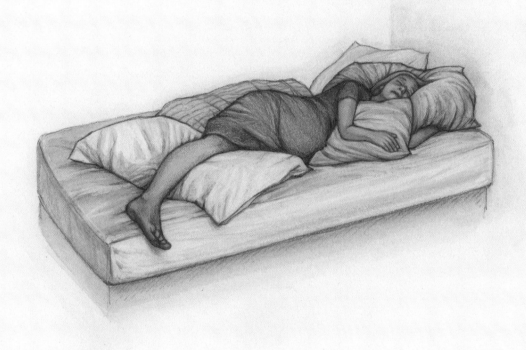

Labor positions often include the abundant use of pillows, which
will ensure the mother's body is comfortable and fully supported.

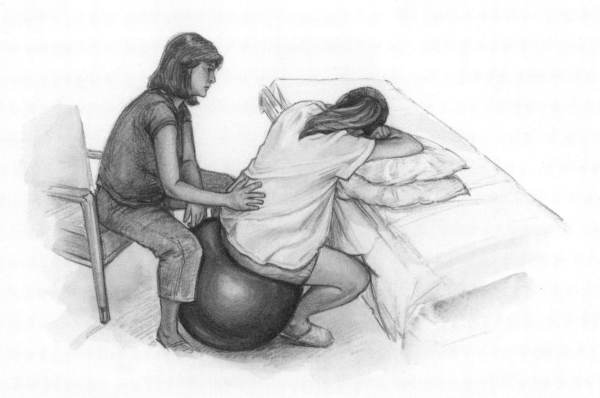

Positions which bring the baby's head down on top of the cervix
will help to stimulate contractions and further labor progress.

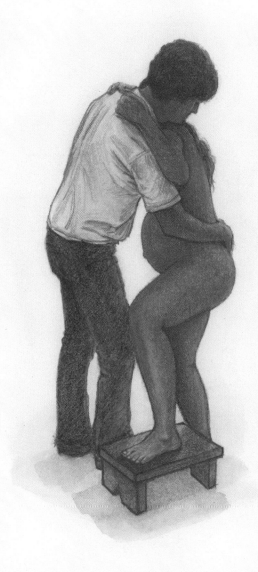

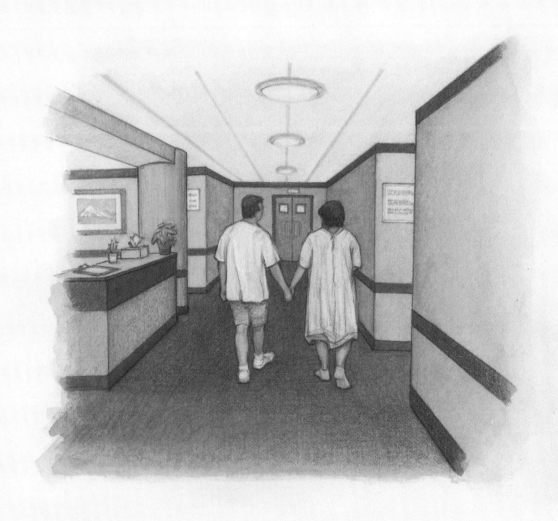

The Importance of Walking

It is important to remember to be active and to incorporate movement in birth rather than remaining in a stationary position.

Walking around during labor will help stimulate contractions and encourage the descent of the baby.

If a contraction begins while you are walking, simply brace yourself against a wall or a labor partner until it is over.

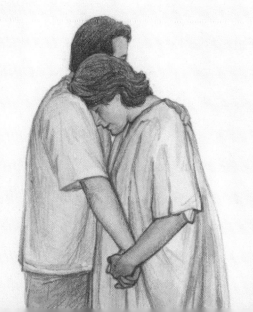

Comfort Techniques

The labor partner can help the mother relieve some of
the physical stress of labor by using comfort techniques.

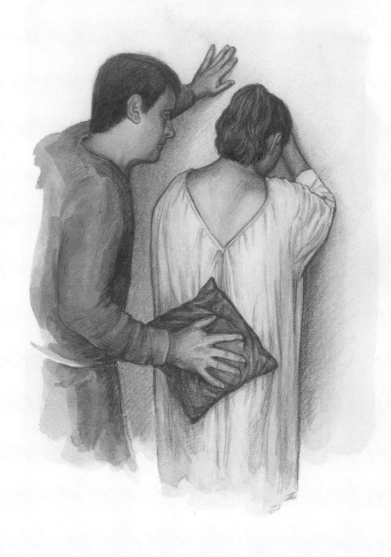

A heat pack can help relieve lower back pain.

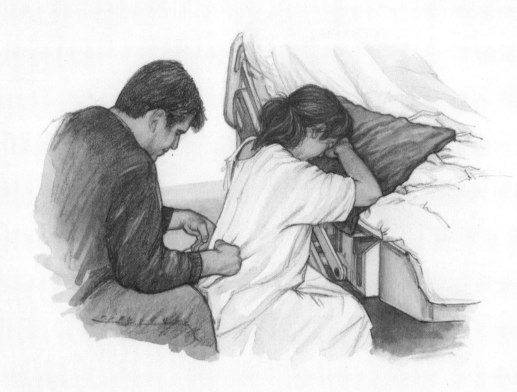

Very firm pressure by a strong hand during a contraction will help relieve
the ache caused by the baby's head coming down through the pelvis.

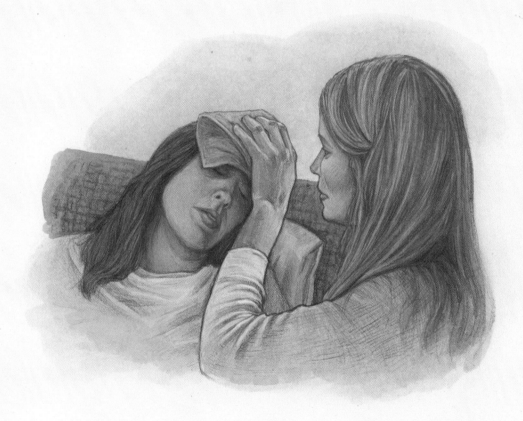

A cool, damp cloth on the forehead helps to soothe the mother and relieve tension.

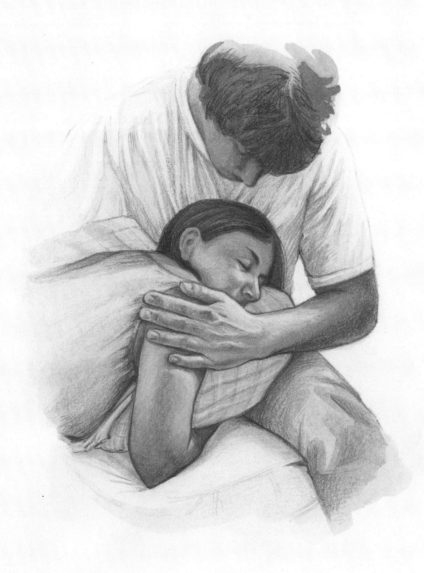

Other areas of tension may include the shoulders, arms and legs.
Here are some additional things that may help:

- light strokes down the arms or legs

- a warm neck pillow around the neck

- massage of the upper shoulders, arms or legs

- a hot bath or shower

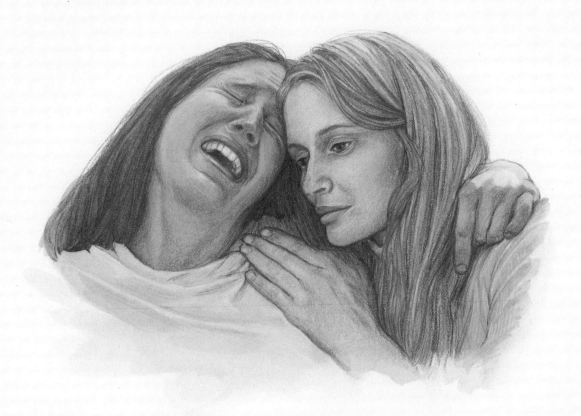

Managing Pain in Labor

When people think of childbirth, they often focus on the pain and on how uncomfortable it is. In fact, they might even mistakenly think that the whole process is a non-stop, painful experience.

The reality is, however, the pain usually occurs only during the contractions. There is rarely any discomfort during the rest periods in between (which are longer than the contractions themselves).

The pain that occurs is caused by both the cervix stretching open and by the descent of the baby through the birth canal.

To manage the pain of labor:

- **Focus on one contraction at a time.** Use your Breathing Techniques, Labor Positions and Comfort Techniques to make it through each contraction.

- **Use your labor partner to guide you through each contraction.**

- **Trust the process.** Trust that your body has the innate ability to deliver the baby and that you are making progress.

How to Move a Woman In Labor

Don't attempt to move a woman while she is having a contraction. Wait until a rest period between contractions to move her slowly and gradually into the new position.

If a contraction begins again while you are moving her, stop and support her there until it is over.

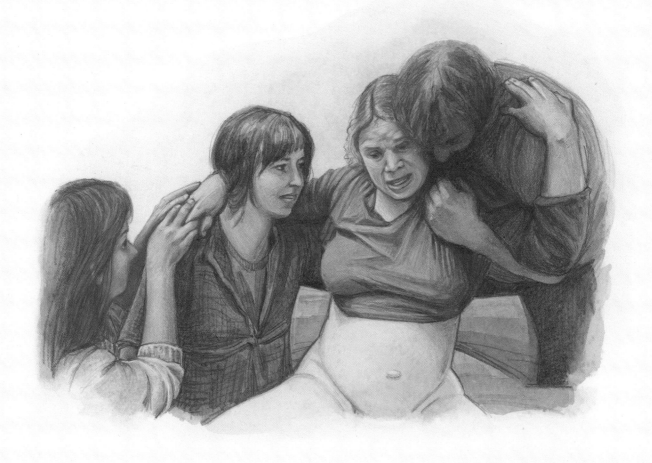

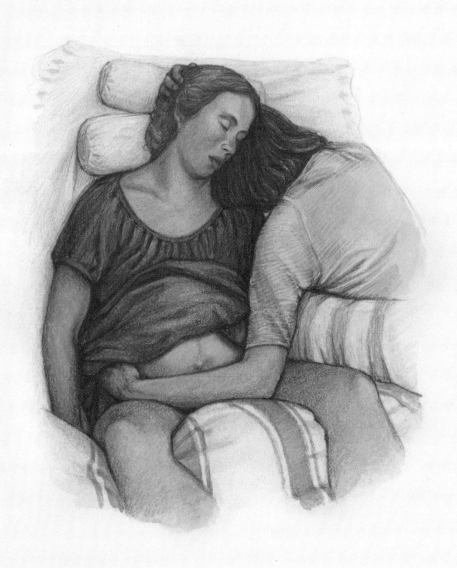

Labor Fatigue

Some labors can be exceptionally long, resulting in a deep exhaustion in the mother.

Labor will continue, however, regardless of how tired she is.

While you can't predict how long a labor will be, you can do your best to be well rested before labor begins.

HOW TO GET THROUGH LABOR

EARLY LABOR

GOALS

- Allow the uterus to dilate the cervix to 4 centimeters
- Arrive at the birth setting when advised by your care provider
- Establish the use of breathing techniques during contractions.

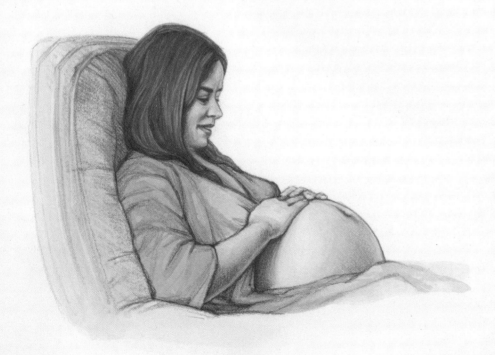

Early Labor is your time to settle into the process at home until you're ready to go to the birth setting.

This is also an opportunity to practice the breathing and relaxation techniques, as it will be the first time to do so under the real conditions of labor.

Contractions are still somewhat mild during Early Labor.

You might take a walk to be outside.

Be sure to stay hydrated and have light meals.

If labor begins in the middle of the night, lie down and rest as much as you are able to.

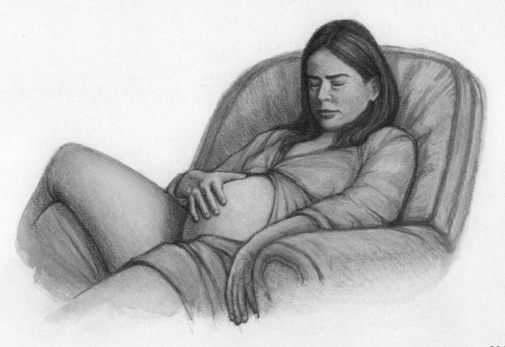

Early Labor Contractions

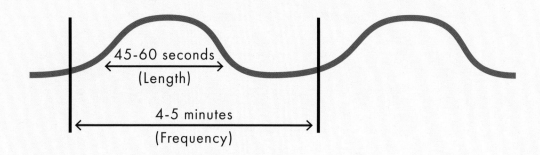

At the beginning of Early labor, the contractions are beginning every 4 or 5 minutes and are lasting between 45 and 60 seconds.

During Early Labor, use the Slow Paced Breathing technique.

Slow Paced Breathing

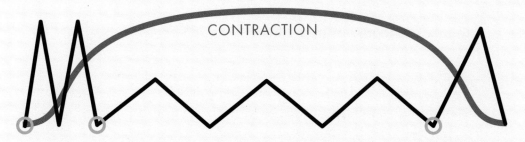

CONTRACTION

1. Begin your contraction with two full breaths in and out.
2. Then use slow, normal abdominal breathing all the way through the contraction.
3. End the contraction with a deep breath again.

ACTIVE LABOR

> GOAL
>
> Allow the uterus to dilate the cervix to 7 centimeters.

By this point in labor, contractions are very strong and consistent. The challenge is to keep from tightening up your body and from fighting the process.

Let go and to let your body do what it needs to do to get the baby born.

This is the time to focus very intently on using your breathing techniques. This, along with the use of labor positions, will get you through each contraction.

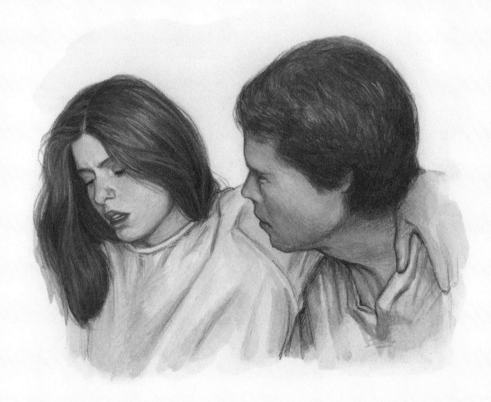

Active Labor Contractions

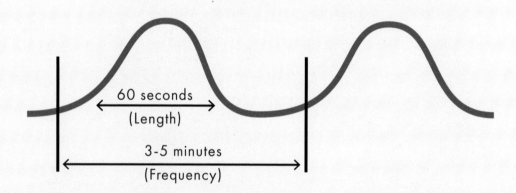

The contractions are now beginning every 3-5 minutes and are about 60 seconds long. The contractions are becoming stronger.

If you are able to, continue to use the Slow Paced Breathing of Early Labor.

Slow Paced Breathing

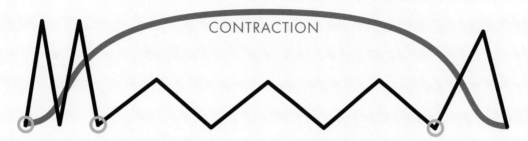

CONTRACTION

1. Begin your contraction with two full breaths in and out.
2. Use slow, normal abdominal breathing all the way through the contraction.
3. End the contraction with a deep breath again.

If you are unable to comfortably use the Slow Paced Breathing, then move to the Moditified Paced Breathing.

Modified Paced Breathing

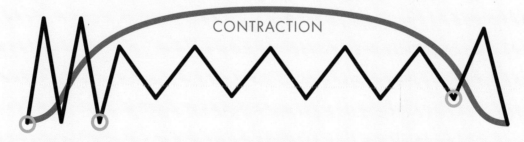

CONTRACTION

1. Begin your contraction with two full breaths in and out.
2. Breathe with slow, half breaths as if to ride over the top of the contraction. Don't try to breathe too deeply. Emphasize the exhale by gently sighing the air out.
3. End the contraction with a deep breath in and out.

TRANSITION

```
GOAL

Allow the uterus to complete the dilation of the cervix
```

Transition is the strongest, most difficult part of labor and requires the greatest amount of focus to get through.

Even though it may feel more difficult to do, continue to use the breathing techniques to make it through each contraction.

Remember to pace yourself so you will be ready for Pushing.

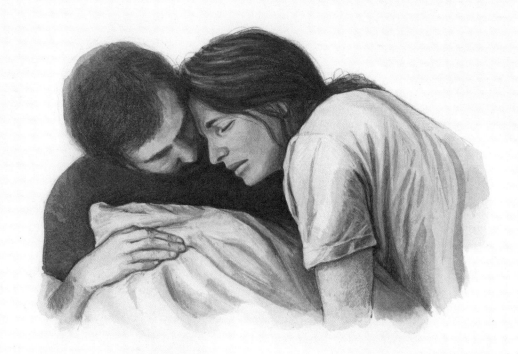

Transition Contractions

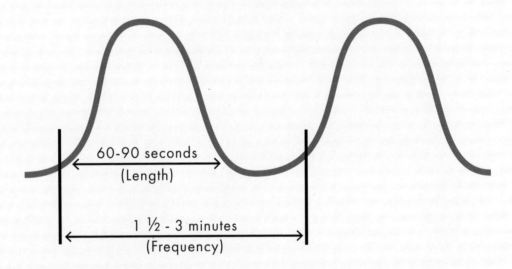

60-90 seconds
(Length)

1 ½ - 3 minutes
(Frequency)

The contractions during Transition will be about 60-90 seconds long and come as often as every 1 ½ to every 3 minutes.

For a gradually progressing labor, continue the
Modified Paced Breathing from Active Labor.

Modified Paced Breathing

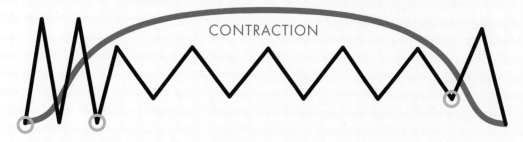

1. Begin your contraction with two full breaths in and out.
2. Breathe with slow, half breaths as if to ride over the top of the
   contraction. Don't try to breathe too deeply. Emphasize the
   exhale by gently sighing the air out.
3. End the contraction with a deep breath in and out.

For a rapidly accelerating labor:

Pant Blow Breathing

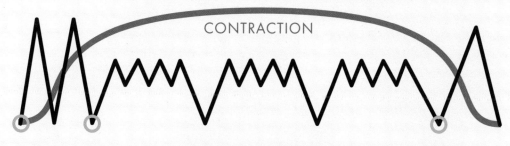

1. Begin your contraction with two full breaths in and out.
2. Take in a medium-sized breath, pant three times and exhale fully.
   Done correctly, this breathing technique has a "hee hee hee whoo"
   sound to it.
3. End the contraction with a deep breath in and out.

The Premature Urge to Push

Pushing should not begin until the cervix is fully dilated and has cleared the baby's head.

Some women, however, will experience an extremely powerful urge to push before this happens. This urge is caused by the baby's head pressing against the rectum.

It is important that the mother not begin pushing until the care provider has confirmed that the cervix is out of the way of the baby's head.

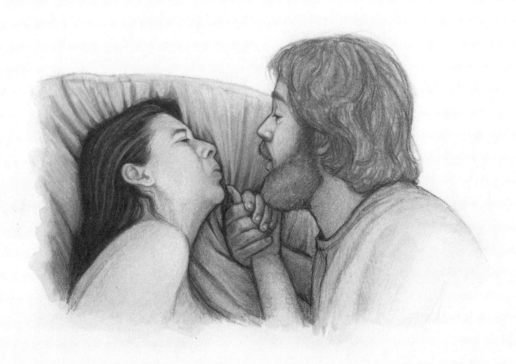

If you are told to refrain from pushing until the cervix
completes its dilation, use the following breathing technique:

Breathing for the Premature Urge to Push

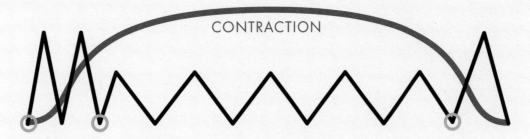

CONTRACTION

1. Begin your contraction with two full breaths in and out.
2. Take a shallow breath in and blow it out forcefully.
   Repeat this shallow breathing for the duration of the contraction.
3. End the contraction with a deep breath in and out.

NOTE: Because of the intensity of contractions at this point, the coach may have to
get in her face and lead her in the breathing technique to keep her from giving in to
the urge to push.

PUSHING

GOAL
Push the baby down the birth canal until it has reached the crowning position

Push as hard as you can during the contraction, then rest until the next one starts.

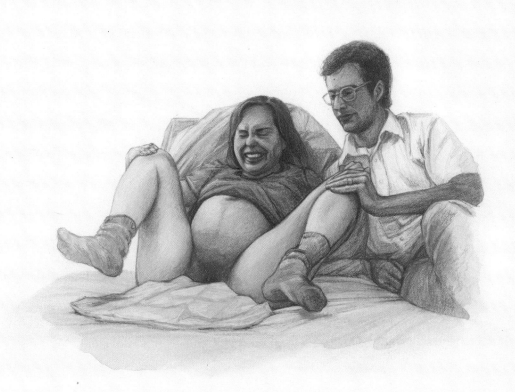

Pushing   Birth   Placenta

Pushing Contractions

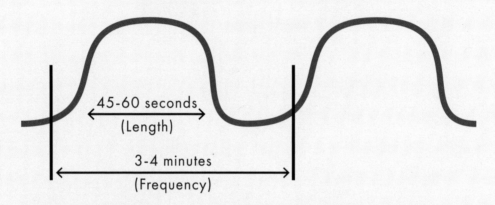

Pushing contractions will last about 45-60 seconds and occur about every 3-4 minutes.

Sustained Pushing

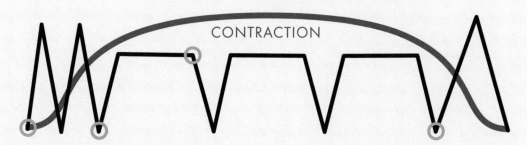

1. Begin your contraction with two full breaths in and out.
2. Breathe in deeply, hold your breath and push as hard as you can.
3. Blow out your air, take a deep breath in and repeat.
4. End the contraction with a deep breath in and out.

If the baby is descending through the pelvis rapidly, the mother will not have to push very hard.   If this is the case, use Modified Pushing Breathing.

Modified Pushing

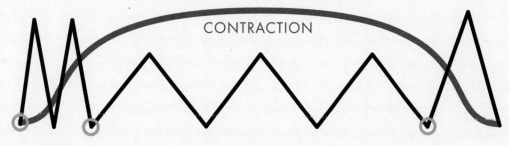

1. Begin your contraction with two full breaths in and out.
2. Inhale and exhale smoothly while letting the contraction do its work.
3. End the contraction with a deep breath in and out.

BIRTH

GOAL
Complete the birth of the baby

Your care provider will guide you in the birth of the baby's head by telling you when to push and when not to push. Follow their instruction while using the breathing for Birth.

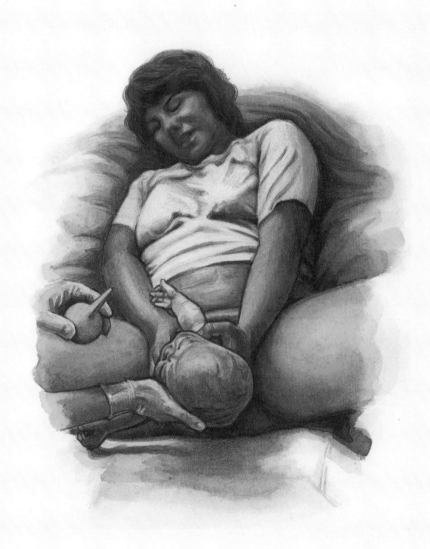

Birth Contractions

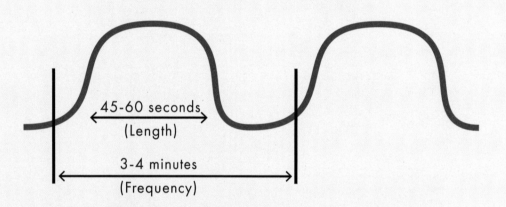

The contractions for Birth are the same as for Pushing.

Birth Breathing

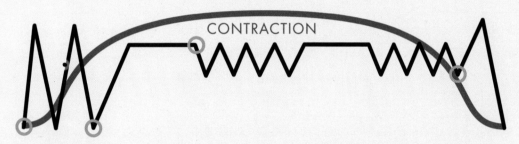

1. Begin your contraction with two full breaths in and out.
2. When instructed to push: breathe in, hold your breath and push gently.
3. When you are told to stop pushing, pant for several breaths.
4. End the contraction with a deep breath in and out.

The Newborn Arrives

> GOAL
>
> If possible, have the baby placed directly on your chest for warm, skin-to-skin contact.

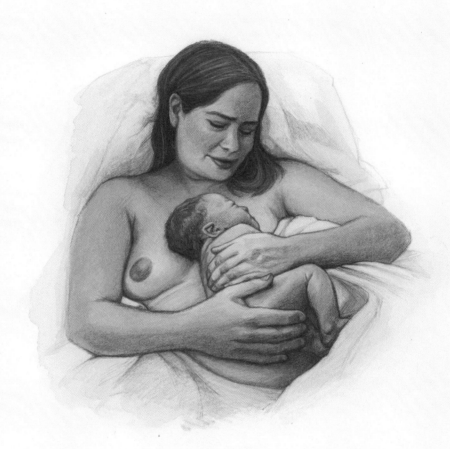

DELIVERY OF PLACENTA

GOALS

- Deliver the placenta

- Ensure the uterus is clamping down and that bleeding is controlled

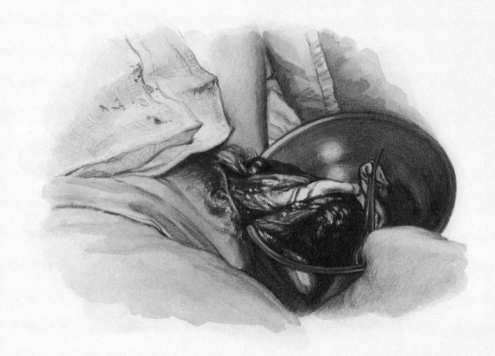

PREPARING FOR LABOR

DESIGNING YOUR BIRTH EXPERIENCE

The birth experience includes three major components.

- **The Birth Environment**
- **The Labor Support Team**
- **Being Prepared**

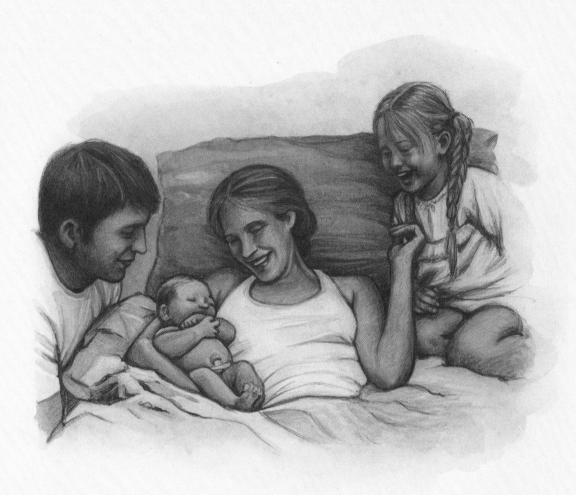

The Birth Environment

The ideal birth environment is one in which the mother can completely relax and focus on the labor process. This should be a gentle and quiet setting for the baby to be delivered into.

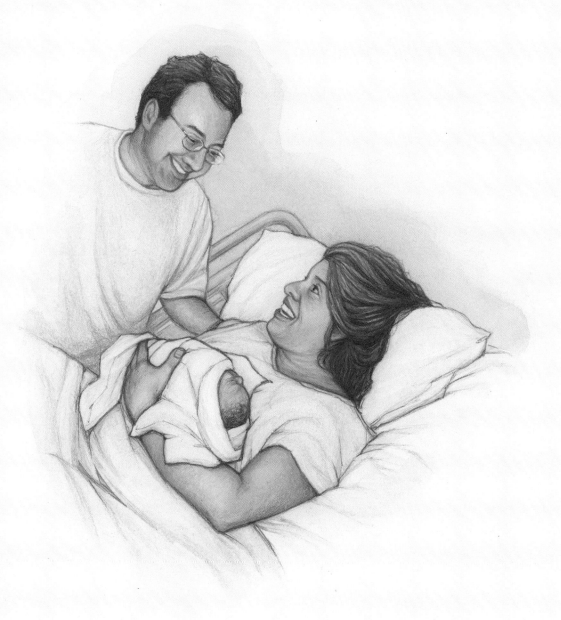

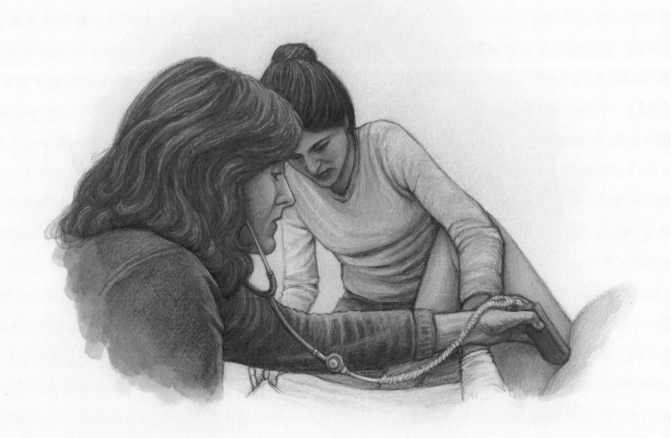

Labor Support Team

Build your labor support team with people who you can trust, who you feel comfortable with and who you believe can best help you get through the labor process. This includes your care provider, medical staff, labor partner or labor coach.

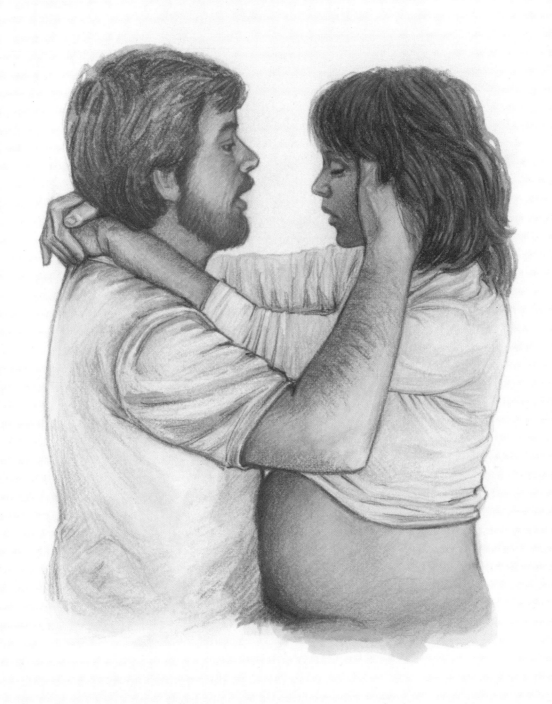

The Labor Coach

The role of the labor coach is to guide, support and encourage the woman through the labor process.

The intensity of the contractions can overwhelm a woman in labor, so she needs someone close by who can coach her through it.

A good labor coach does the following:

- **Observe.** The coach will observe what the woman is experiencing and anticipate what is coming next.

- **Understand.** The coach needs to understand what is happening well enough to provide appropriate and helpful guidance. This understanding is achieved by knowing the labor process and the tools to get through it.

- **Support.** The coach must be a stable source of emotional and physical support so that the laboring woman can relax into the process.

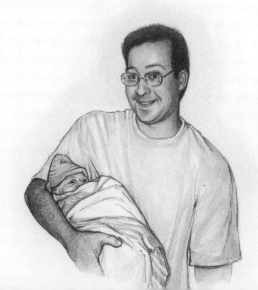

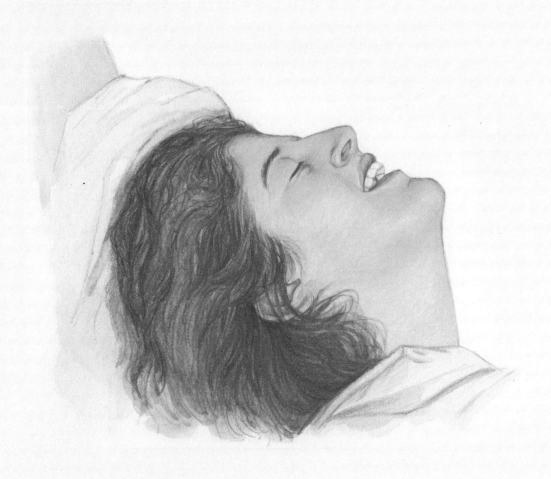

Being Prepared

You can't go back and do your birth again. You have one opportunity to make it the best experience possible.

Ultimately, having a baby is a woman's personal journey of self-discovery. No one can do this process for her.

You cannot predict how a birth is going to go. All of the steps can be taken, however, to ensure she has the support she needs to do her best.

Being prepared is being educated on the birth process, knowing the labor techniques and having a good team in a good environment.

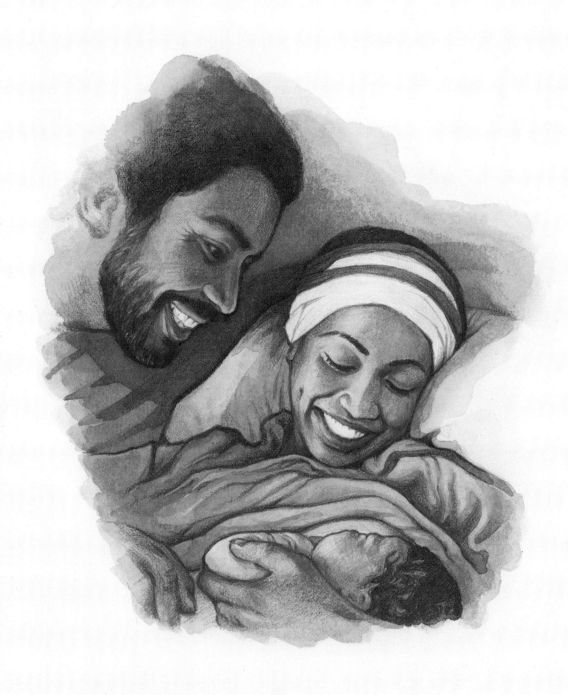

Creating Your Birth Plan

A birth plan is a written description of the goals of your labor and of how you would like to manage the process.

It's helpful to use your birth plan when choosing your care provider and birth setting.

During the labor, this birth plan will inform the medical staff of how you would like to treat your birth process.

The goal of the birth plan is to coordinate everyone to work together.

THE BIRTH EXPERIENCE

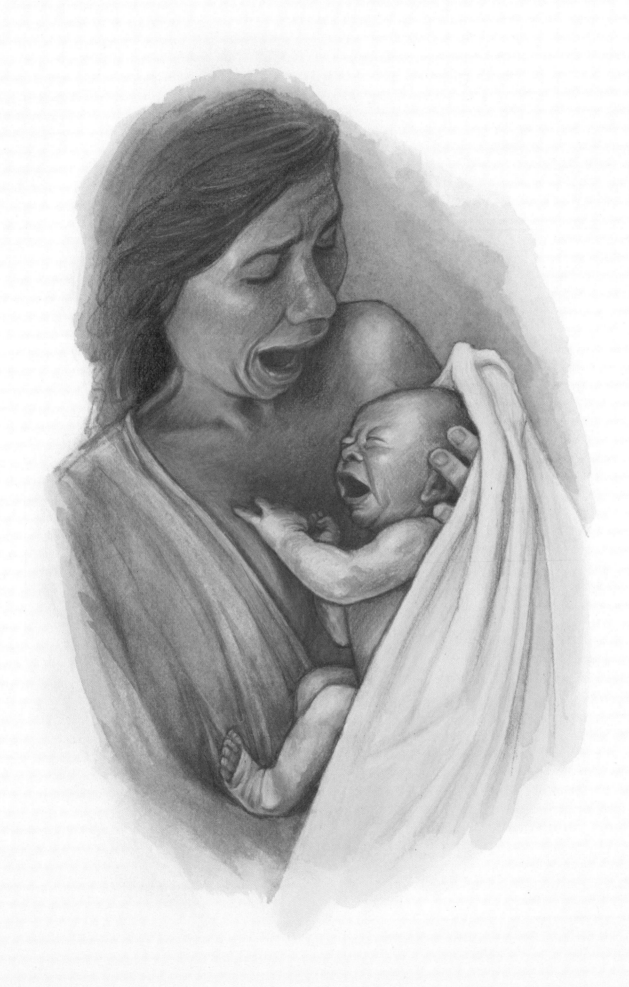

Childbirth is not just a physical experience;
it has a deep emotional impact on everyone involved.

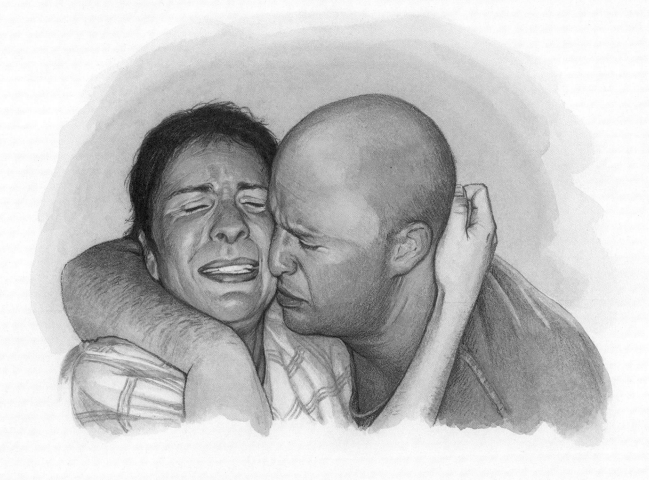

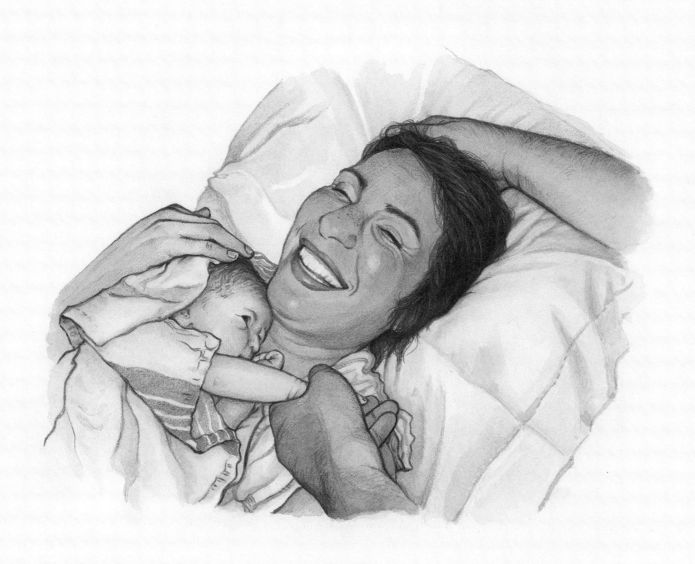

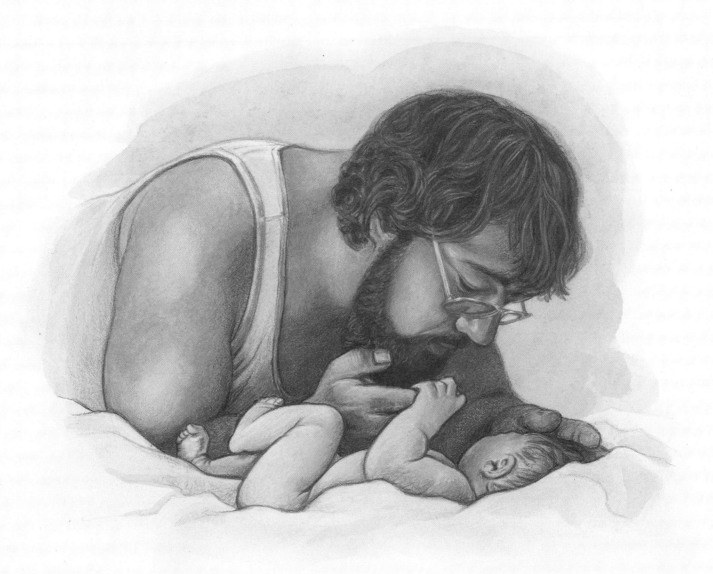

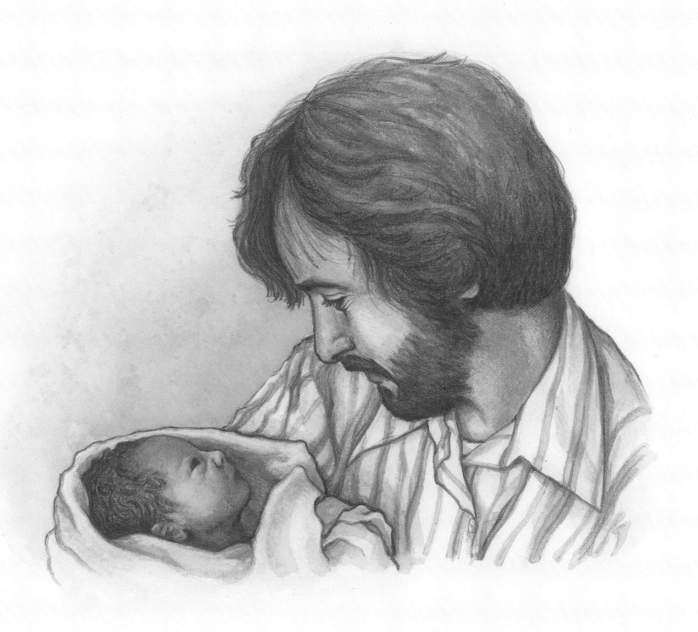

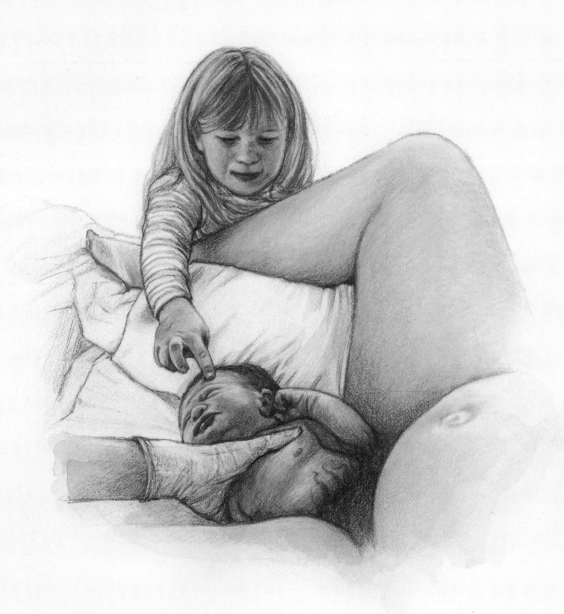

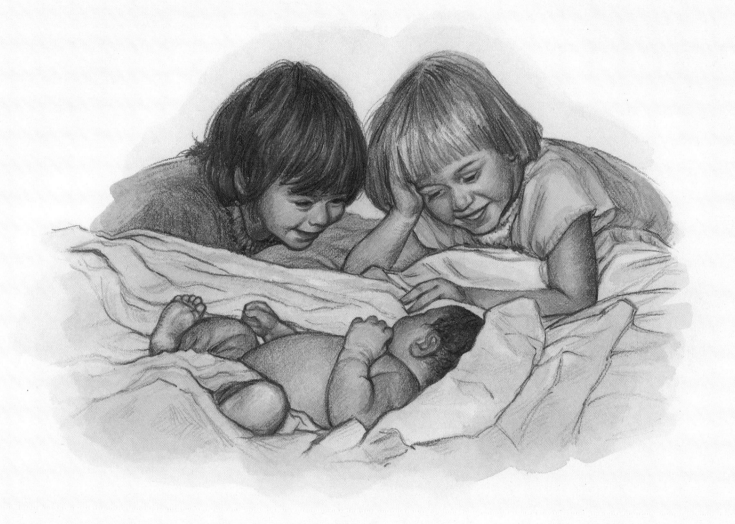

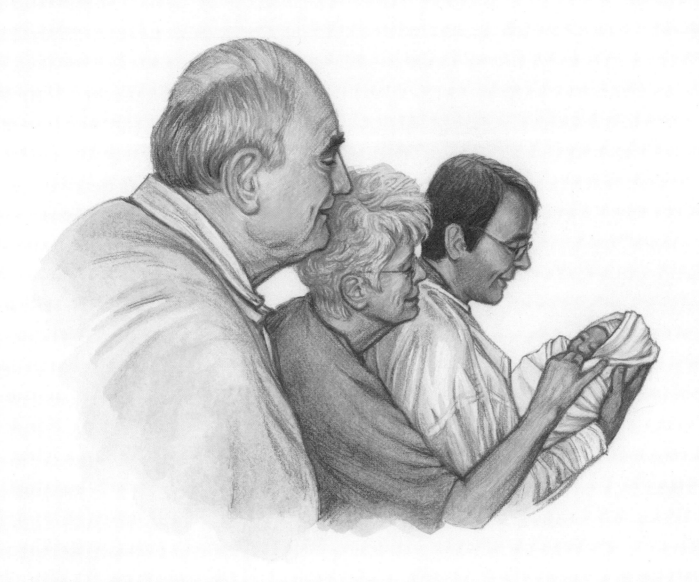

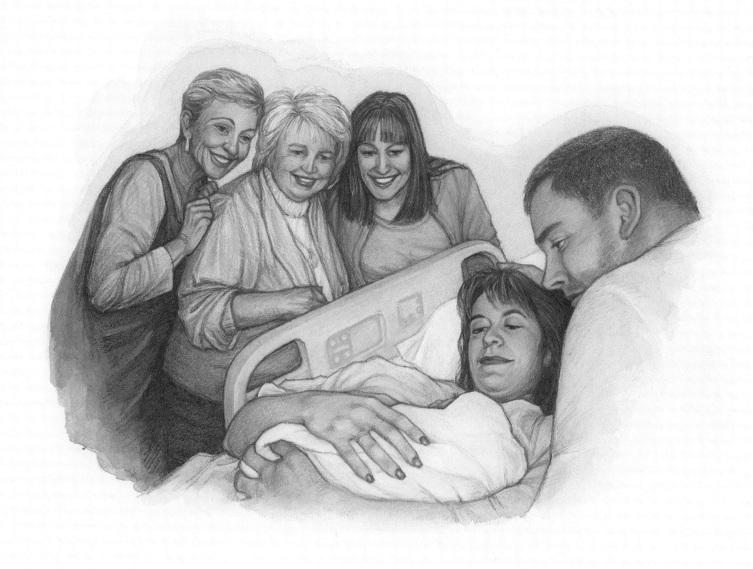

In fact, the impressions from this experience, pleasant or unpleasant, are carried for a lifetime.

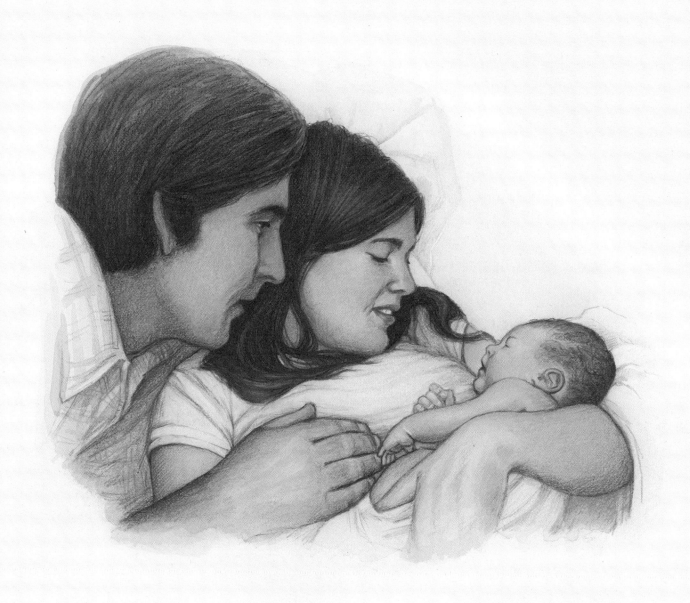

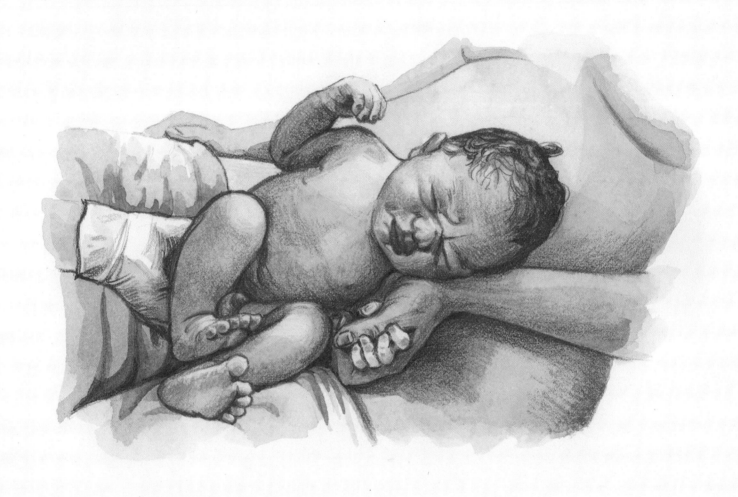

The powerful effect of this birth experience on the newborn can be observed in his or her appearance and mood in the time following birth.

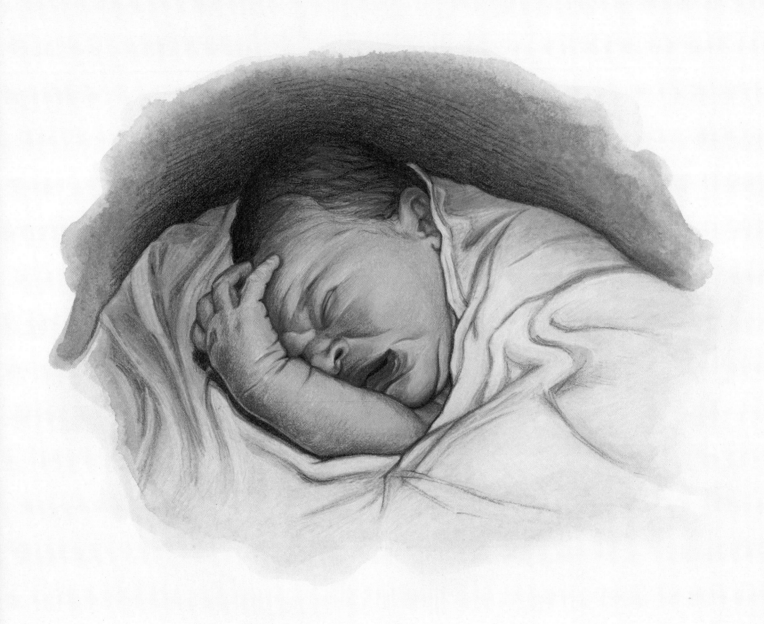

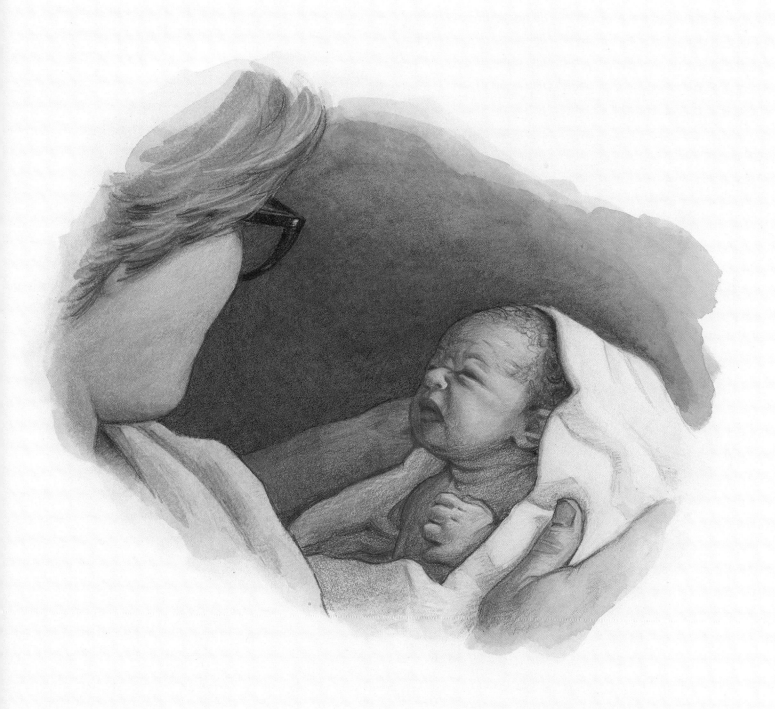

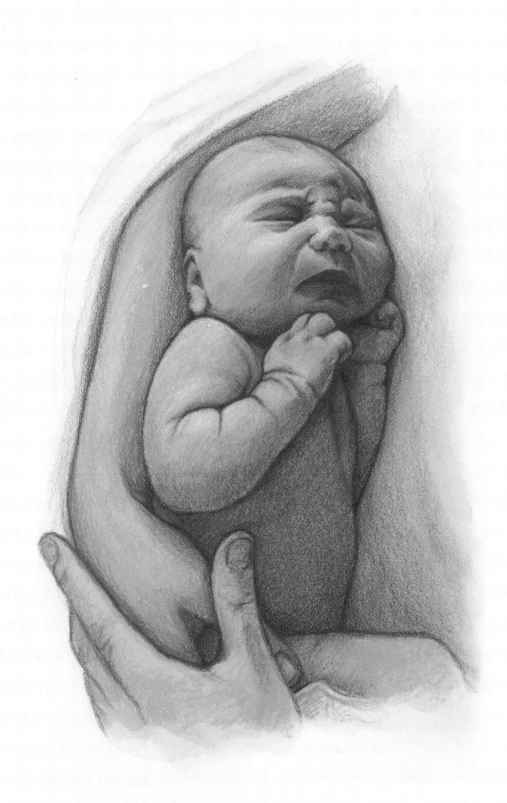

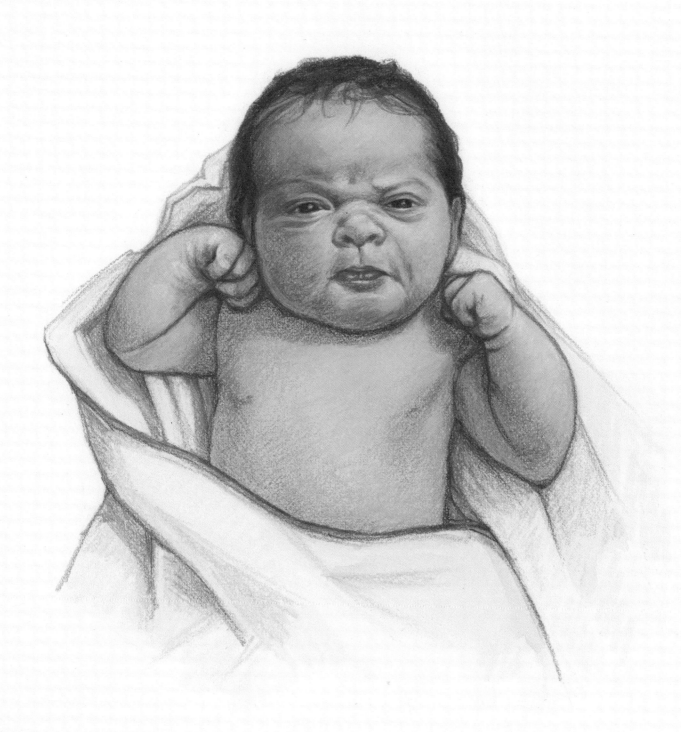

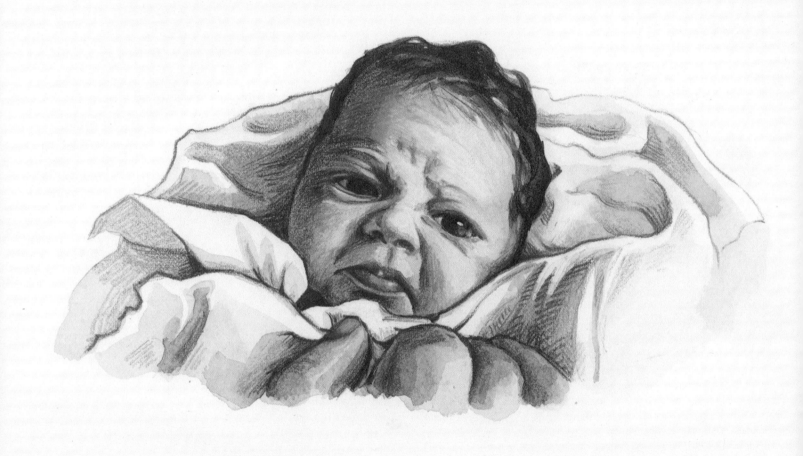

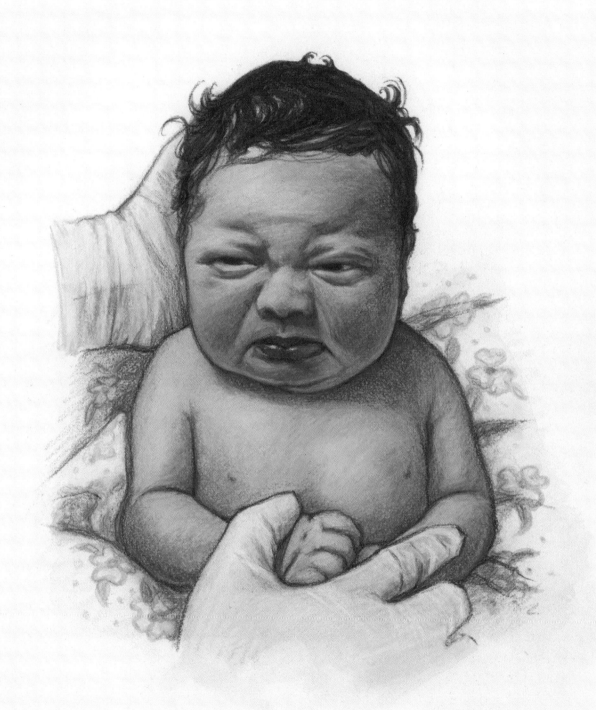

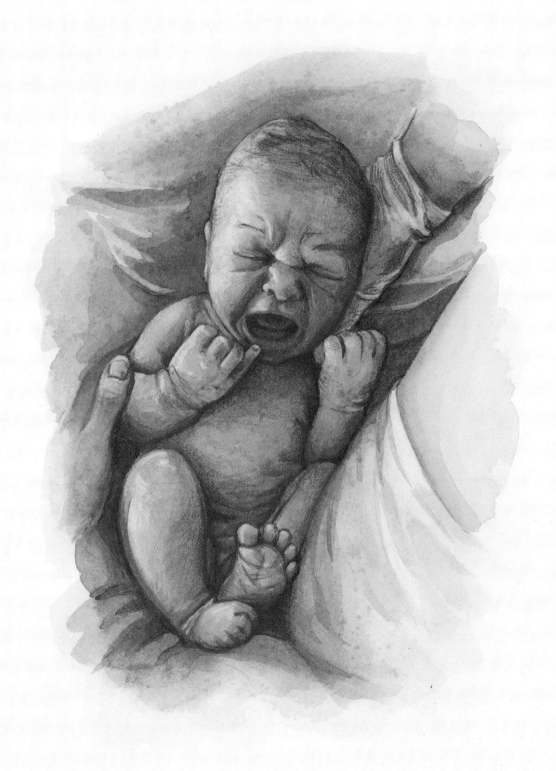

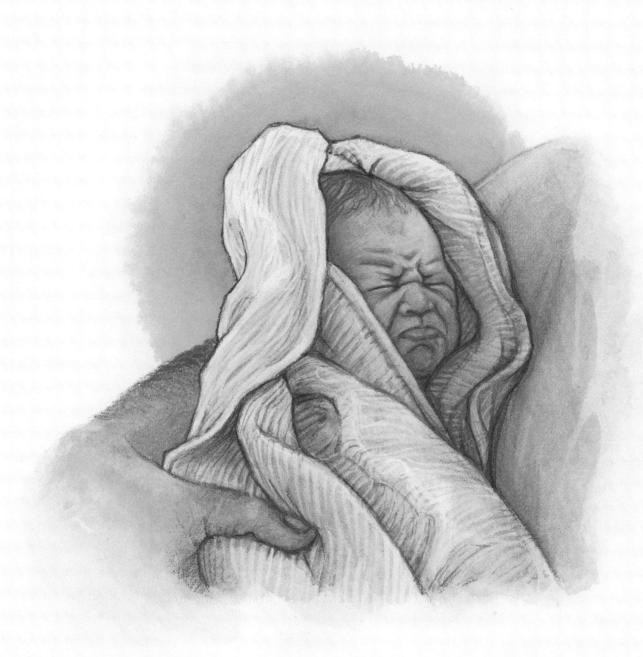

The time of your newborn's birth is the moment to welcome a new person into your family.

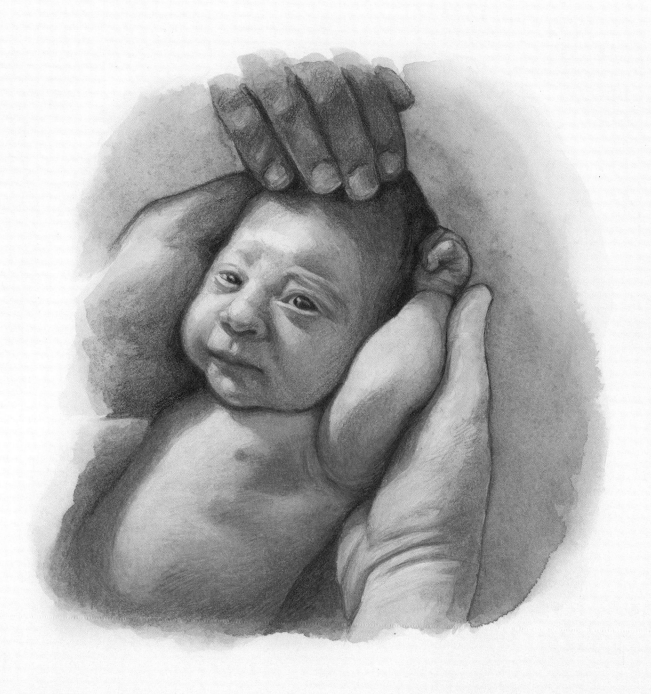

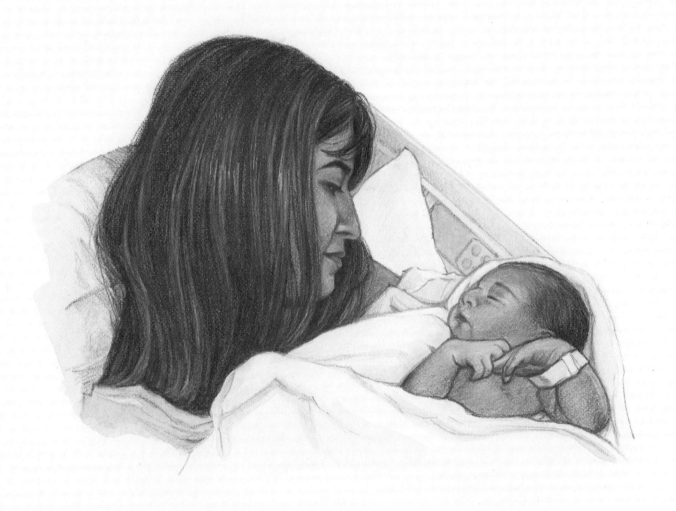

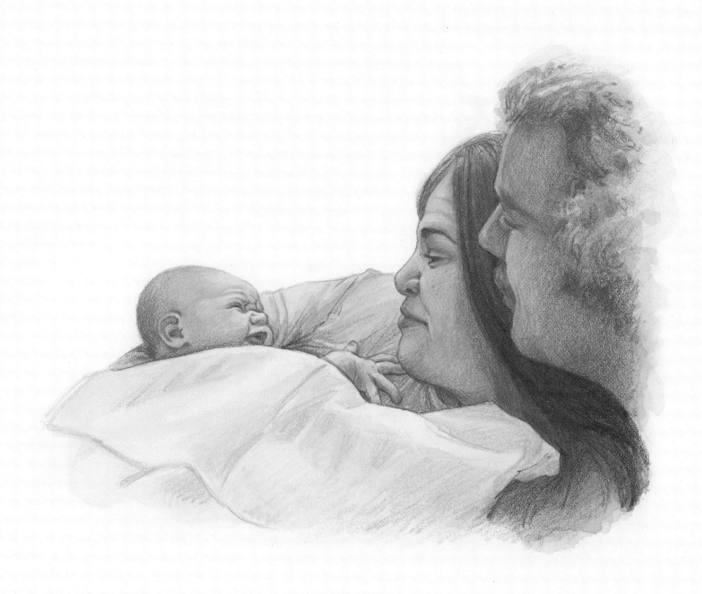

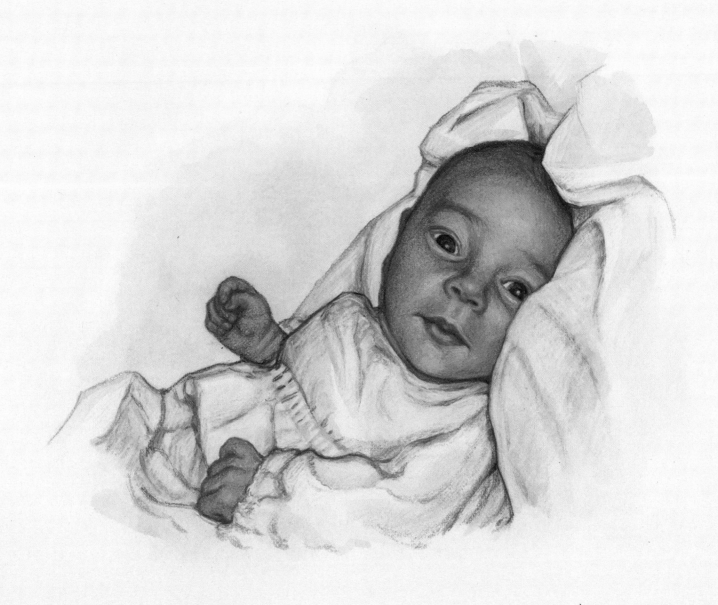

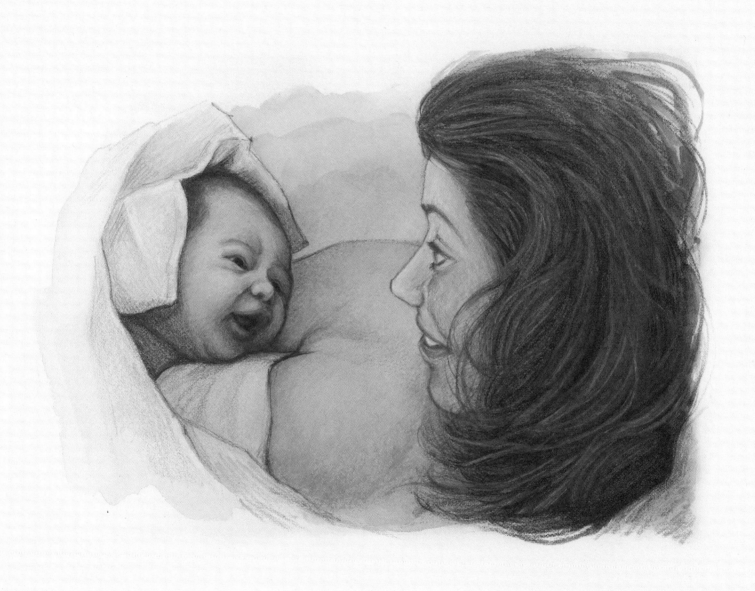

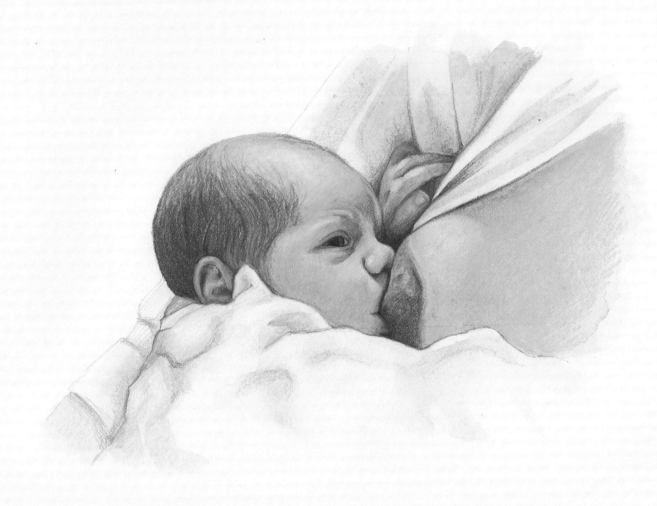

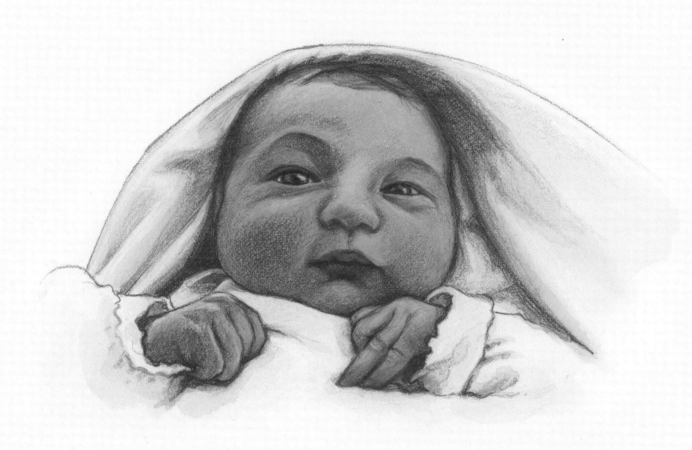

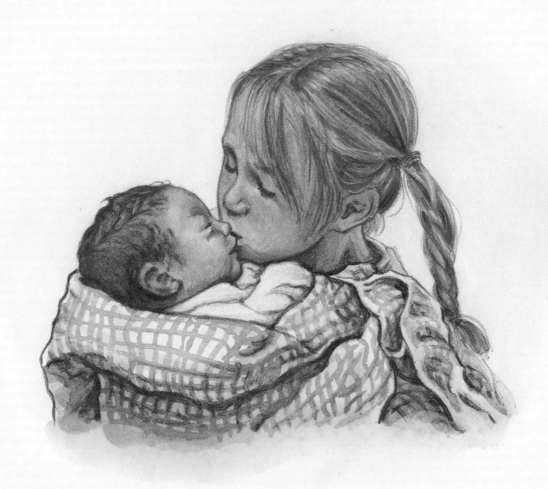

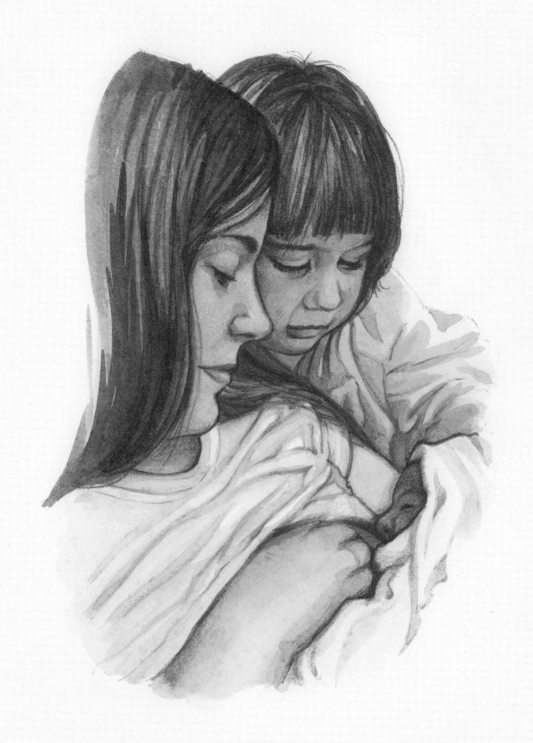

CLOSING COMMENTS

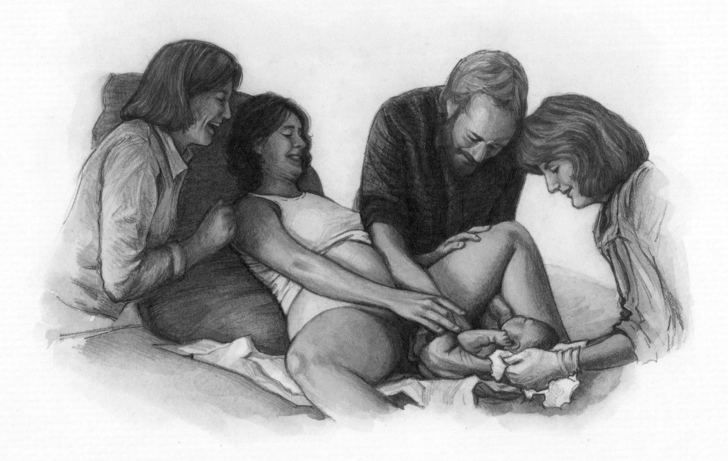

My journey of 30 years of being a midwife ends with this book.

This now becomes your journey.

Use this information to make your own birth a memorable one.

"I don't teach a woman how to have a baby;
I help her remember."

Heather Moll

MOTHERHOOD

It's the lifeline that connects us to those who came before

It's the way we create those who come next

It's bringing a person safely into this world,

and it's caring for them until they are able to care for themself

It's persevering through any obstacle to meet my baby for the first time

It's being prepared so that when labor begins I know what to do.

by Jeremy Moll

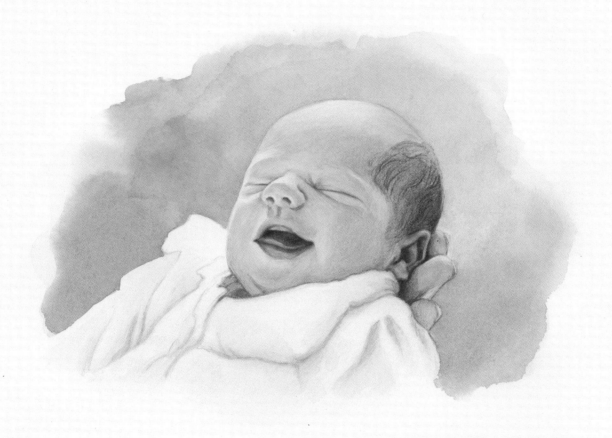

ADDITIONAL RESOURCES

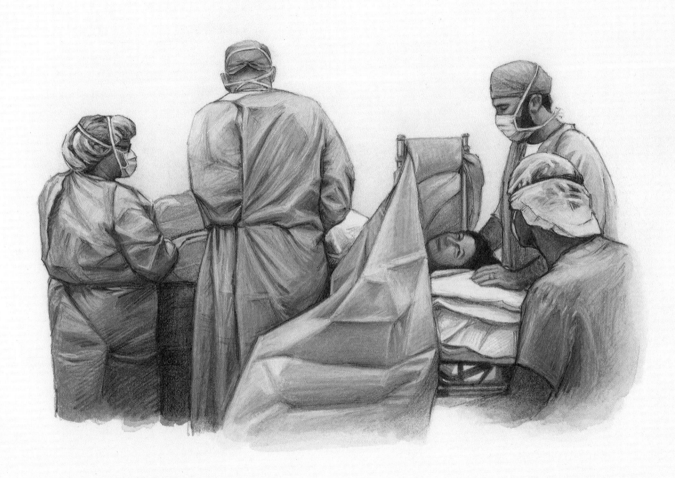

MEDICAL INTERVENTION
When Mother Nature Needs a Helping Hand

This book outlines the natural process of childbirth. The reality is, however, that some births depart from this natural process. In those instances, a carefully managed intervention may become necessary.

It is important to understand what is being recommended by your care provider and to know what your choices are.

Here are some of the questions you can ask.

- What is the departure from the normal birth process?

- How will this departure affect the birth?

- What medical procedure is being suggested?

- What are the pros and cons of this procedure?

- Are there any alternatives to this procedure?

- Is it possible to have more time to see if the labor works itself out?

Taking the time to understand the situation will allow you to continue your participation in the management of the labor.

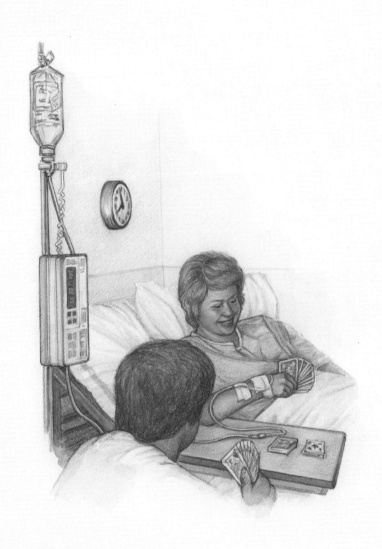

Labor Induction

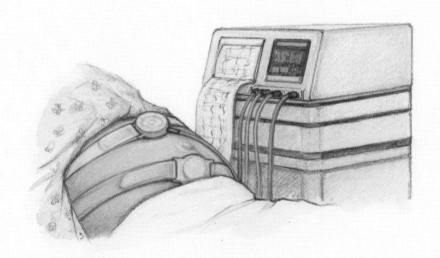

Fetal Monitor

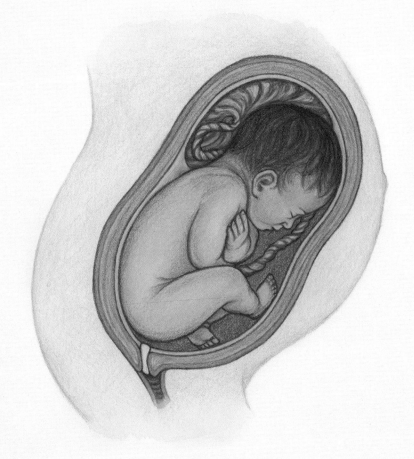

Breech Position

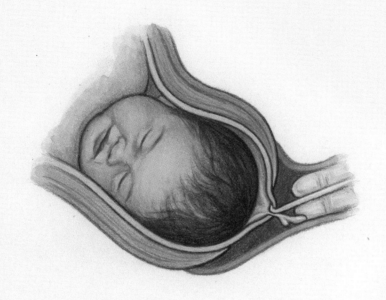

Membrane Rupture

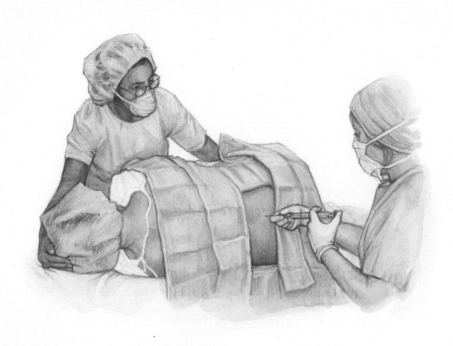

Epidural

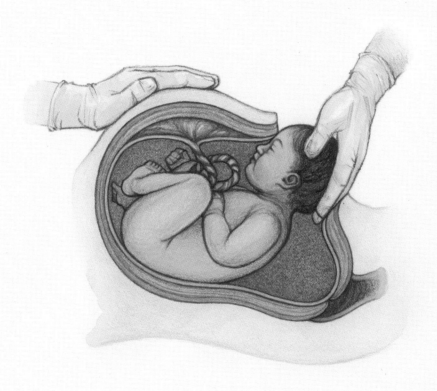

C-Section

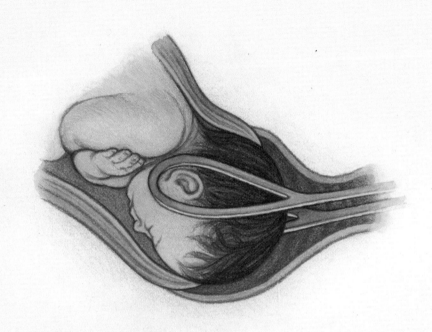

Forceps Delivery

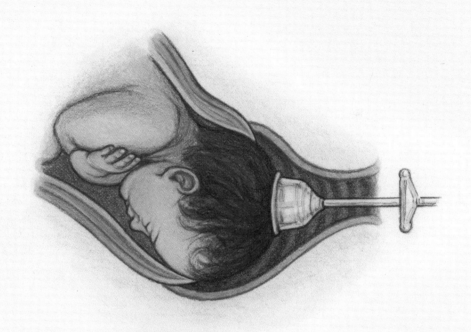

Vacuum Extraction

SUMMARY OF BREATHING TECHNIQUES

FIRST STAGE OF LABOR

Slow Paced

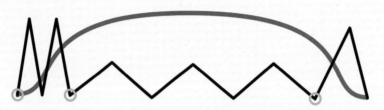

1. Begin your contraction with two full breaths in and out.
2. Then use slow, normal abdominal breathing all the way through the contraction.
3. End the contraction with a deep breath again.

Modified Paced

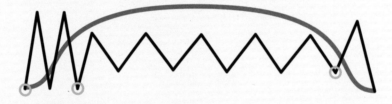

1. Begin your contraction with two full breaths in and out.
2. Breathe with slow, half breaths as if to ride over the top of the contraction. Don't try to breathe too deeply. Emphasize the exhale by gently sighing the air out.
3. End the contraction with a deep breath in and out.

Pant Blow

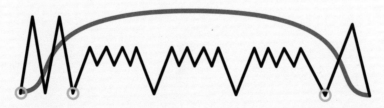

1. Begin your contraction with two full breaths in and out.
2. Take in a medium-sized breath, pant three times and exhale fully.
3. End the contraction with a deep breath in and out.

Keep From Pushing

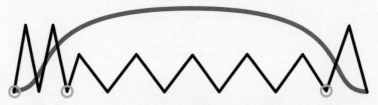

1. Begin your contraction with two full breaths in and out.
2. Take a shallow breath in and blow it out forcefully.
3. End the contraction with a deep breath in and out.

SECOND STAGE OF LABOR

Sustained Pushing

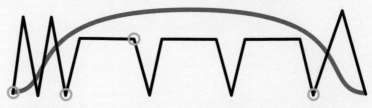

1. Begin your contraction with two full breaths in and out.
2. Breathe in deeply, hold your breath and push as hard as you can.
3. Blow out your air, take a deep breath in and repeat.
4. End the contraction with a deep breath in and out.

Gentle Pushing

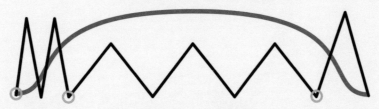

1. Begin your contraction with two full breaths in and out.
2. Inhale and exhale smoothly while letting the contraction do its work.
3. End the contraction with a deep breath in and out.

Birth

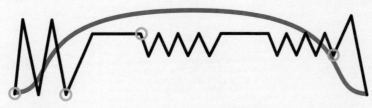

1. Begin your contraction with two full breaths in and out.
2. When instructed to push: breathe in, hold your breath and push gently.
3. When you are told to stop pushing, pant for several breaths
4. End the contraction with a deep breath in and out.

SUMMARY OF LABOR POSITIONS

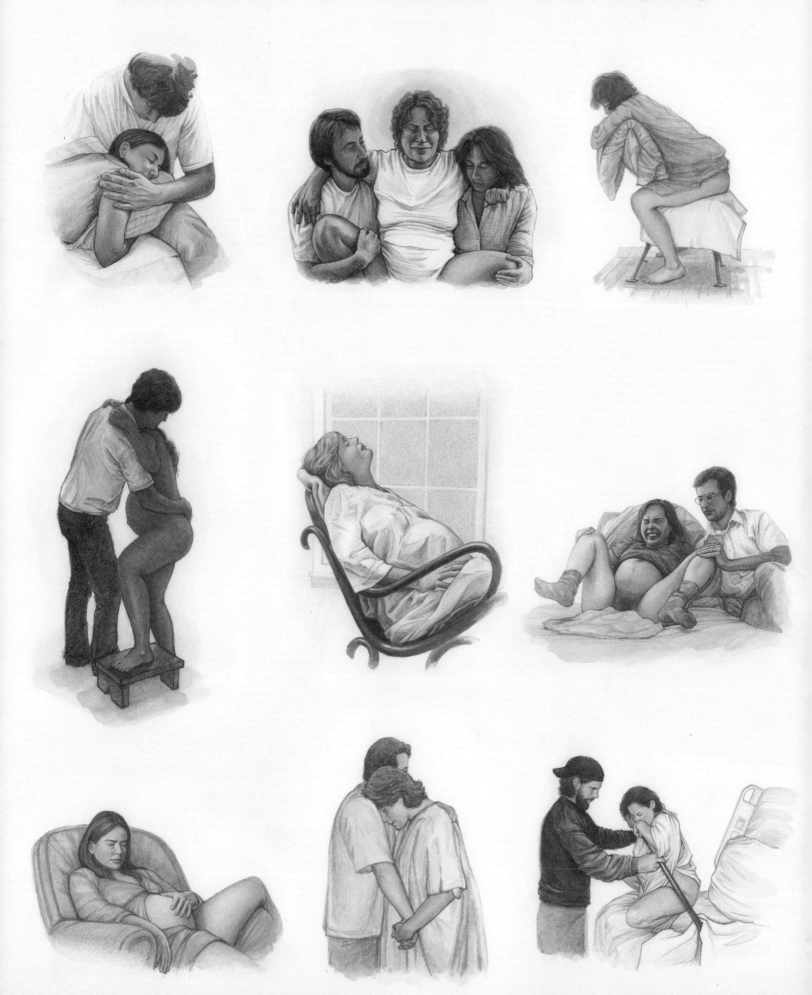